managing chronic pain

Also by Dr Vandana Prakash and Dr Mary Abraham

Conquering Pain: How to Prevent It, Treat It and Lead a Better Life

managing chronic pain

DR VANDANA V. PRAKASH
DR MARY ABRAHAM

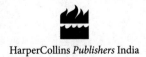

HarperCollins *Publishers* India

First published in India by HarperCollins *Publishers* 2024
4th Floor, Tower A, Building No. 10, DLF Cyber City,
DLF Phase II, Gurugram, Haryana – 122002
www.harpercollins.co.in

2 4 6 8 10 9 7 5 3 1

Copyright © Dr Vandana V. Prakash and Dr Mary Abraham 2024
Diagrams courtesy Dr Mary Abraham

P-ISBN: 978-93-5489-910-2
E-ISBN: 978-93-5489-939-3

The views and opinions expressed in this book are the authors' own and the facts are as reported by them and the publishers are not in any way liable for the same.

This book is not meant to be used to self-diagnose or treat any medical condition. For diagnosis or treatment, please consult your own physician. The authors and publishers are not responsible for any needs that may require medical supervision and specifically disclaim any and all liability arising directly or indirectly from the use or application of any information in this book. Practising anything in this book by readers is done at their own risk. References are provided for informational purposes only and do not constitute endorsement of any website or other sources.

Dr Vandana V. Prakash and Dr Mary Abraham assert the moral right to be identified as the authors of this work.

All rights reserved. No part of this publication may be reproduced, stored in a retrieval system, or transmitted, in any form or by any means, electronic, mechanical, photocopying, recording or otherwise, without the prior permission of the publishers.

Typeset in 11.5/15.2 Adobe Garamond at
Manipal Technologies Limited, Manipal

Printed and bound at
Nutech Print Services - India

This book is printed on FSC® certified paper
which ensures responsible forest management.

To
Our patients

'Healing is more about accepting the pain and finding a way to peacefully coexist with it. In the sea of life, pain is a tide that will ebb and weave, continually. We need to learn how to let it wash over us, without drowning in it. Our life does not have to end where the pain begins, but rather, it is where we start to mend.'

Jaeda DeWalt

Contents

Foreword ix

Preface xi

1. Transition from Pain to Chronic Pain — 1
2. Decoding Chronic Pain — 15
3. Chronic Pain and the Mind: The Indivisible Phenomenon — 42
4. Risk Factors for Chronic Pain — 69
5. Physical and Psychological Impact of Chronic Pain — 95
6. Assessment in Chronic Pain — 125
7. Managing Chronic Pain — 144
8. Integrated Rehabilitation Management: A Case Discussion — 189

Acknowledgements 209

Glossary 211

Notes 215

Index 217

The detailed notes pertaining to this book are available on the HarperCollins *Publishers* India website. Scan this QR code to access the same.

Foreword

You must read *Managing Chronic Pain*. You don't have to be a medical person; you are a human being, and that is reason enough.

The American psychiatrist Dr Elisabeth Kubler-Ross described a pattern in how we deal with bad news or grief. The first is denial, the reaction: 'This cannot be true'. Next comes anger. Unfortunately, the disease or pain is not embodied in front of you to shout at, and so the anger gets directed at those closest to you. Then you go on to bargaining—this often takes the form of offerings to God in return for a cure or flitting from doctor to doctor or from one system of medicine to another. Depression follows, which in some cases can be so bad that the person loses the perception of what it takes to deal with life.

And finally, comes acceptance. Now you confront the problem, accept what you cannot change, and seek out the best possible course of action to deal with what can be changed. Thus, minimizing damage and getting on with life.

These reactions hold true for all of us in the society. Somewhere deep inside, we know that disease and disability may disrupt every life some time or other; but we choose to not think about it. 'Doctors and nurses will deal with it when the time comes,' we think. But the problem is that the conventional medical system we know of can only deal with the disease. When the disease cannot be cured, particularly in India, the healthcare system often rejects the person. Or it continues to see only the disease, ignoring the interaction between mind and body, choosing not to see the social destruction of the person, and pretending not to see his/her spiritual death.

The first of the four noble truths that Buddha taught was: 'All beings experience pain and unhappiness as part of life.' This is more true for those who live with chronic pain. If we all live in denial of the pain, we have no way of dealing with it when it does happen to us or to a loved one. Then illness, pain or suffering can destroy us socially and emotionally. But if we are in acceptance, we can be prepared to confront the issue, and minimize suffering through appropriate action.

Life is certainly full of suffering for people living with chronic pain, who may be around five million in India. This book will help us understand the problem, to give a hand to hold to those who suffer from chronic pain, and to make their life as liveable and enjoyable as possible.

Remember, it is not about *them*. Someday, we or our loved ones could be *them*.

Dr M.R. Rajagopal
Chairman, Pallium India
Director, WHO Collaborating Centre for Training and
Policy on Access to Pain Relief

Preface

Human beings are no stranger to pain, it has always been a part of our existence. Yet, despite this long association and day-to-day experience with it, the history of pain itself has been a long and, often, chequered one. It took centuries for pain to be extricated from the realms of morality and religion to be recognized as a biological phenomenon and a few centuries more for it to be understood as a biopsychosocial one.

Pain is an experience that all living beings encounter during their life span. It is an exceedingly unpleasant condition to be in, although certain types of pain have a protective function. While acute pain is sudden and recent in onset and tends to get alleviated faster, chronic pain and cancer pain behave like a tedious gate that never stops creaking. Unlike acute pain, it has no protective value but instead brings a host of psychological, social and even spiritual pain in its wake. In fact, chronic pain is a disease in itself.

Chronic pain is understood as pain that has lasted for more than twelve weeks and has persisted long after the healing period or inflammation is over. Instead of the beneficial function it is supposed to serve, physical pain gets overshadowed by a significant overlay of psychological and social factors. This heralds the onset of chronicity, which leads to untold misery and suffering and adversely affects the quality of life of the individual. It then intrudes into the lives of the afflicted persons and brings with it, a myriad of problems in the personal, familial, societal and occupational domains.

Psychologically speaking, a chronic pain patient is often found to be depressed, anxious, stressed and harbouring thoughts of self-harm or suicide. It impinges not only the patient's life, but also affects those who are closely associated with them. When a person is distressed, it reflects in their relationships with their spouse, family and friends. Performance at the workplace gets affected too, which can belie any happiness, sense of satisfaction or fulfilment.

People afflicted with chronic pain are often not able to reconcile to the fact that besides medical treatment, they need psychological management in order to overcome their distress and get well. In most cases, the patients are not even aware that the mind can be the dominant factor in perpetuating their pain and suffering. This is a challenge that most clinicians face. Explaining chronic pain using the biopsychosocial model is, therefore, imperative before any management programme can be implemented. Patients need to understand the complexity and interplay of various biological and psychosocial facets that are instrumental in developing, maintaining and even in acting as barriers to a successful treatment.

Accordingly, a thorough assessment of the patient is done from the physical point of view, followed by a detailed psychosocial assessment. The latter involves understanding the person's personality, prior adjustment, ability to adapt to situations, coping with stress, presence or absence of social support and the cultural milieu in which the person has been brought up. Given the increasing number of patients who could be categorized as chronic pain patients and the plethora of predicaments they are faced with, such as their deteriorating health, crippling medical expenses with economic repercussions, litigations, breakdown of family ties and increased societal burden, one can appreciate the serious ramifications that chronic pain incurs medically, socially, personally and financially. This reiterates the significance and need to address psychosocial issues in the overall management of chronic pain.

Keeping these important issues in mind, this book has been written in consonance with the biopsychosocial model of pain. Hence, chronic pain and its treatment have been discussed in a holistic manner in the eight chapters of this book.

Chapter one describes a case study as well as introduces important concepts related to pain, total pain and how pain becomes chronic.

Chapters two and three decode the physical and psychological aspects of chronic pain. In chapter two, we highlight how pain is currently viewed, how it is perceived and what classifies it as chronic. Chapter three is devoted to understanding how our thinking processes, distorted thinking, emotionality and social reasons gain importance in leading to the chronicity of pain. The focus of these chapters is to understand the nuances and ramifications of chronic pain, the profound effect it has on the psyche of a person and how the mind affects the very sustenance of chronic pain. It explains to the reader how chronic pain and the mind are two sides of the same coin.

Chapter four is dedicated to elucidating the modifiable and non-modifiable risk factors that can cause chronicity of pain. Chapter five talks about the impact chronic pain has on a patient's life, which encompasses the physical, psychological, familial and occupational changes that take place for the sufferer. Chapter six focuses on the role that assessment of chronic pain plays in implementing an appropriate treatment programme. Chapter seven offers a comprehensive view of the multi-modal and multi-disciplinary treatment options available for a person with chronic pain. Chapter eight describes how an integrated rehabilitation programme can be beneficial and the ways by which various therapeutic techniques are interwoven to work in tandem to bring relief from pain and improve the quality of a person's life.

When we came up with the idea for this book, the world was still living through the Covid-19 pandemic. So we felt it was only relevant to incorporate the effect it had on chronic pain. The consequences of lockdowns and working from home on the ergonomics of the working class, the increased workload due to non-availability of household help during the pandemic and the lack of physical exercise as people were wary of venturing outdoors and the long-term effects of Covid-19 infection had contributed to a deterioration in the physical and mental health of people. That, in turn, had led to many instances of new onset of chronic pain and even worsening of pre-existing chronic pain. To add to that, fear of the virus had prevented people from visiting pain clinics, many of which had to be temporarily suspended in order for healthcare personnel to, instead, focus on treating victims of the pandemic.

This book is primarily for the non-medical public. To make it reader-friendly, we have incorporated several case studies, which have been discussed from a biopsychosocial perspective, so that the importance of a holistic approach gets highlighted. The emphasis is on multi-modal rehabilitation in order to alleviate all facets of chronic pain. Since mental processes very often overlay the physical aspects in chronic pain, this book has been written for you to understand how best to decrease disability and improve the overall quality of life from a holistic point of view.

1

Transition from Pain to Chronic Pain

The tap-tap-tap of the stick made me look up. I saw through the glass door a man trying to manoeuvre the bend in the corridor and at the same time trying to straighten his back. He slowly approached my chamber door. Since my chamber is divided into two rooms, I can see the patients from a distance even before they enter the inner sanctum. The slight stoop of his shoulders and deeply lined face spoke of silent suffering, but his radiant skin belied his age. I guessed that he was still in his mid-thirties. The expression on my face prompted him to say rather enigmatically, 'Doctor, I'm destiny's child!'

Settling himself slowly and gingerly with a little ostentatious fussing in the chair, he gave me a rather boyish smile. It seemed as if the years had rolled by and I was seeing the younger version of the person in front of me. I opened the conversation with my usual questions for self-introduction. 'Later,' I said, 'I would like to understand the cryptic remark you made when you entered my room.'

His name was Rahul. He was thirty-four years old, married and had a three-year-old son. He had graduated as an engineer and then did a management course. He belonged to a business family, in which the other shareholders were his father, one paternal uncle and three unmarried paternal aunts. Among the five siblings, Rahul was the only surviving child. His uncle's daughter had died two years ago during childbirth. He mentioned that since he and his cousin were the only children in such a large and affluent family, both had been doted upon by everyone. 'In fact,' he added, 'you can say, I had five mothers and two fathers. Needless to say, I was thoroughly spoilt as manipulating the elders was easy.'

'Since money was never an issue, I led an extravagant lifestyle and would spend lavishly. I can easily say that my existence was larger than life. So from a very young age, sometime in my early teens, I started experimenting with alcohol and later with drugs in the company of my friends. For me, education was not really a priority since I had the reassurance that whether I studied or not, I would ultimately join my family business and one day inherit everything.'

'Did anyone try to stop you or at least try to guide you?' I queried.

'My mother did try, but my aunts, uncle and father would not allow her to reprimand me.' He sat ruminating for a while and then, looking up, said, 'Perhaps, my mother was the only one who genuinely and selflessly loved me. I realize it now and try to make it up to her.

'Anyway, under the influence of alcohol and drugs, I met with several accidents. One rather major accident happened almost eight to nine years ago, when I was trying to ride my friend's new motorbike. Being unfamiliar with the new mechanism, I had crashed into the railings of the road divider as I could not control the bike. My leg got trapped under the bike, badly smashing my left kneecap [patella] and fracturing my left shin bone. I had to undergo a knee and leg surgery to set it right. I remember suffering a lot of pain immediately after the surgery. Gosh! Those days were terrible when they first tried to make me ambulate following the surgery. I used to dread each physiotherapy session because it was so painful. But my protests and pleadings fell on the deaf ears of the doctors, nurses and physiotherapists.

'After getting discharged from the hospital, my parents had arranged for physiotherapy sessions in a nearby clinic. I had to continue those dreadful sessions for both pain relief and rehabilitation. It was at this point that my friends persuaded me to try alcohol for pain relief. I was told that it would deaden my pain and, frankly, it was easier and more enjoyable. I foolishly fell for this idea—and on the pretext of going to the physiotherapy clinic, I would go to my friend's place during the time of the supposed session and have a booze session instead.

'My parents were puzzled that despite undergoing expensive physiotherapy and meeting the best orthopaedic doctors, I was neither relieved of pain nor was I able to walk without support. It had been four months since the surgery and the pain had only become worse. I was unable to carry on with my daily activities and even my sleep cycle was disturbed.

'It was at that point that I decided to mix drugs with alcohol as I thought that would give me some respite from pain. I did not,' he said contemplatively, 'pause for even a moment to think where I was heading and neither did my "adviser" friends.

'When my family came to know what I had been up to, they thought that marriage was the only solution to make me a more responsible person.' He smiled ruefully and continued. 'Well, I don't think it generated any wisdom or responsibility in me because I continued with the booze parties. That lifestyle continued for several years, even when I became a father. The birth of my son brought no change in me or my way of life. My friends and I considered ourselves too young to shoulder such responsibilities, which we would anyway be bearing in the years to come.

'Now let me tell you what happened on that fateful day. Ravi, one of my friends, had just announced that he would no longer be attending those parties. We were surprised at first, then angry with him. After badgering him for an explanation, he told us that his wife had given him the ultimatum to choose either his friends and booze or her. He told us with a determined look that he had decided to choose his wife and seven-month-old daughter. This statement of Ravi's sobered all of us and realization dawned that we were only wrecking our lives with our foolish and reckless behaviour. Spontaneously and with one accord, the rest of us also decided to get on the same bandwagon as Ravi.' Rahul then paused in his narrative, looked at me and, smiling faintly, asked whether I was familiar with the word 'bandwagon'. When I nodded, he continued.

'I believe we were all sincere in our resolve to turn into a new leaf. As a token of our resolution, we decided to go home sober for once. But the little imp in us was not entirely subdued by our seemingly monumental decision. For old times' sake and to more or less say farewell to our old lives, we hit upon the idea to go to Munna Chacha's dhaba for tea. This dhaba was near our college gate. While parting to get into the two cars between us, I suggested that we race to the dhaba. The others unanimously agreed, with bets also being placed as to who will win the race.

'All I remember is that Ravi and I were in the same car, and I was driving fast at about a speed of 120 km/h. Three of our friends were close behind in the second car. I do not know what exactly happened, all I can recollect is that their car rammed into ours. I still remember the sickening sound of metal-on-metal crunching and grating, followed by explosive sounds. Doctor, that sound still haunts me in my dreams,' he said rather despairingly. Distress was writ large upon his face.

After a long pause, he continued, 'I woke up in hospital with severe pain, after being in coma for three days. I was told that I had fractured my pelvic bone [hip bone] and left femur [thigh bone]. My left shoulder was also dislocated and my left forearm was fractured.

I had to undergo surgery once again, but this time it was for my left thigh bone and left forearm. I had to wear a sling for my dislocated shoulder and was advised complete bed rest for the pelvic bone to heal. It was a very traumatic period for me. My wife and mother were constantly at my bedside caring for my every need. Doctor, the pain stuck to me closer than a brother, casting deep shadows in my life. Despite analgesics, every slight movement was painful. I remained in hospital for two months. After I was discharged, although I was able to hobble around with a walker, the pain was still unbearable.

'I had asked several times about the welfare of my friends but was told evasively that they were in different hospitals and nothing much was known about them. After coming home, I slowly gathered that I had lost three of my friends in the accident. The fourth friend, Ravi, had sustained severe head injury and was now in a comatose state. I have not visited him yet.' He suddenly covered his face with his hands as tears trickled down from it slowly. I waited for him to regain his composure.

'I'm responsible for the death of my friends and for Ravi's state,' he spoke despondently. This was perhaps indicative of survivor's guilt in him. I asked him to elaborate on it further. He continued in this vein, 'It was I who had suggested the race in the first place. Had I not done so, this tragedy would not have happened, and that too when we had decided to turn a new leaf. I don't think we were racing to have tea. Rather, we were racing for death and destruction. And I lost, hands down.' Saying this for the first time, he looked squarely into my eyes with despair and grief. 'Now, do you believe I'm destiny's child?'

Since the accident eleven months ago, he had been in and out of hospital for the first three months—his main problem being chronic and unrelenting pain in his shoulder, low back, hips and thigh that was not responding to analgesics. He had been referred to a pain specialist, but he had refused it because he felt that pain was a punishment that he must bear for all his misdeeds. In fact, he even justified pain as a form of penance and a sentence from God that he must undergo. It was singularly evident that he carried immense guilt and still lived with the emotional trauma of the accident, suggesting spiritual pain along with physical and psychological pain. Since he could not carry on with his work and family dynamics were also affected, social pain, too, was evident. He often felt that he should join his deceased friends as there was no point in living with so much pain. He even had suicidal thoughts, although he neither planned it, nor made any attempt to do so.

At this point I asked routine questions to check for other psychopathologies. Rahul's responses indicated that he had been suffering from depression, severe guilt feelings, visible and palpable anxiety about succumbing to alcohol as a means to cope with his feelings and chronic pain. Since movement caused considerable pain, he also had anxiety about any kind of treatment that forced him to exercise or be active. He said he was very vigilant when his son came near him as he had to adjust his stiff and painful legs to accommodate the child climbing on to his lap. On being asked what had motivated him to come in for treatment, as history suggested an otherwise attitude towards medicines and therapies, Rahul confessed that since he was wary of his son's playful behaviour, the child often felt that his father did not love him. Moreover, he had observed that his paternal aunts were being overindulgent towards his son as they were towards him in his formative years. He wanted his wife to concentrate more on the child rather than him, so that history does not get repeated. He wanted his son to grow up as a dependable and trustworthy human being.

It was important to know a little more about his family, particularly his wife—as to how she was coping with the circumstances at home. Here again was a bittersweet situation. He admitted, 'I'm never left alone and my whole family take turns to be with me. They all try to be sickeningly cheerful, and the accident is never discussed. Even when I try to broach the topic, it is always skilfully manoeuvred to other neutral topics.' I then tried to gauge the couple's relationship, to which he replied, 'The nurse in her has overtaken the wife, but she remains the best mother to my son.'

In the end, he looked at a piece of paper and said that he had to meet two other people that day—the head of the pain clinic, Dr Mary Abraham, and the head of the physiotherapy department. I directed him to Dr Abraham.

At the Pain Clinic

My first impression of this gentleman as he walked into my clinic was of a stooped and dejected-looking man walking with a limp and not quite making eye contact with me. Dr Vandana had already apprised me of his medical history, and I knew that I needed to be cautious and subtle in my approach with him especially while taking his history. His wife and mother accompanied him and I requested all of them to take a seat and get comfortable. Initially, he was hesitant but gradually he grew more confident and told me all about his accident, his past surgeries, his turbulent postoperative course and his problem with chronic pain and disability. His left shoulder was painful and that had led to restriction of his left arm's movement. The back of his head and forehead ached as well. His lower back, hips and buttocks were tender and painful to touch. His left hamstrings were very tight and hurting so much that he was not able to take his full body weight on his left leg. The pain in his shoulder was moderate to severe and the pain in his lower back and hips was severe. His back pain would get worse on standing, walking and even getting up from the sitting position. In fact, every movement was pure agony.

He mentioned he was unable to find a comfortable posture at night and that disturbed his sleep. He usually woke up feeling tired and unrefreshed in the morning, along with a headache. Although he was taking analgesics round the clock, it was not giving him enough relief. Only massage and hot fomentation were giving him some respite. He told me that although he used to take alcohol and drugs until the accident, for nearly a year now he had been off those substances.

Physical examination revealed numerous tender areas on his left shoulder, lower back and buttocks. He had severe muscle spasm in these areas as well as his left thigh, as revealed by taut and tight muscles. Range of movement of his left shoulder was limited. Examination of the X-rays revealed normal alignment of his dislocated shoulder, pelvis, left forearm and left thigh bone—all of which suggested good bone healing.

It was apparent to me that the pain was primarily myofascial in origin and was affecting not only his day-to-day living but the very quality of his life. The chronicity of pain had stemmed from numerous factors, which included insufficiently treated postoperative pain, extensive injuries and inadequate rehabilitation. But there was more to it than just the physical aspects as revealed by his psychosocial history. There were dominant psychological, emotional, social and spiritual factors that were compounding the chronic pain condition.

I explained to him the biopsychosocial nature of pain and that it is not just a physical experience but an amalgamation of psychological, social and cultural factors. To explain it better, I led him and his family near the charts put up in my chamber depicting various aspects of chronic pain.

The first chart showed the potential factors that play a crucial role in the pain experience. I explained to them that since our body and mind are not separate entities but two sides of the same coin, when there is disturbance in one it will affect the other. Therefore, both the pain experience and recovery from pain are a biopsychosocial phenomenon. This chart also clearly showed various biological

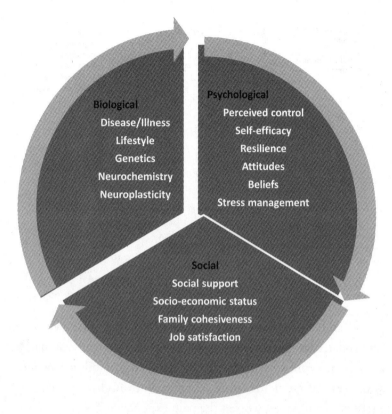

Fig 1.1: Biopsychosocial model of pain experience

factors that can lead to chronic pain and how our mind and social environment influences it. At their nod, indicating that this was understood, I took them to the second chart.

At this point, I explained to them about the concept of 'total pain' and that pain is not just an unpleasant physical experience. A person having physical pain, especially if it is chronic, suffers varying degrees of emotional pain, social pain and even spiritual pain. Physical pain could be due to cancer, injury, inflammation, age-related degenerative changes and central sensitization syndromes. As explained earlier, when pain tends to be persistent, then psychological and social

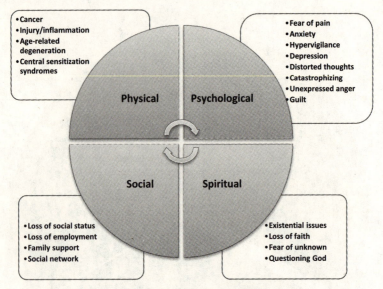

Fig 1.2: Total pain concept

factors and, at times, even spiritual factors become intertwined and inter-related to the pain experience. Psychological pain can manifest as anxiety, depression, hypervigilance, anger, irritability, frustration and even suicidal ideation. Distorted thoughts, particularly catastrophizing ones, worsen the pain experience. Social pain could be fear of dependency, role reversal, loss of social status, financial difficulties, lack of family support and strained relationships, loss of employment and so on. Then there is spiritual pain in some people. Spiritual pain is experienced when a person feels abandoned by God, struggles to understand the meaning of life and pains borne, difficulty in seeking or giving forgiveness or worst of all, losing hope and faith in God.

So you can see that chronic pain is not just physical in nature but a combination of psychological, social and even spiritual factors.

As I proceeded to the third chart, which depicted how chronic pain causes physical and mental deconditioning, Dr Prakash entered the pain clinic.

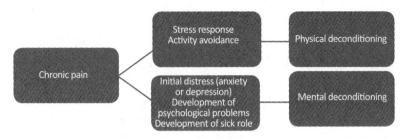

Fig 1.3: Chronic pain: Physical and mental deconditioning

We explained the terms 'physical' and 'mental deconditioning' and how both occur as a result of chronic pain. Physical deconditioning, I told Rahul, occurs as a result of the stress response and pain behaviour such as fear avoidance. I went on to further elaborate these terms so that he could understand it better.

Pain, especially if it is chronic, is a potent stressor and elicits the stress response through the hypothalamic-pituitary-adrenal axis, which is part of the endocrine system. The prolonged increase in steroid hormones (cortisol levels) in our circulation due to the stress response can have a negative effect on the body. This is because steroids help to generate glucose that is required for mobilizing the stress response. But this occurs at the expense of breakdown in protein, which results in weakness of muscles, bones and nervous tissues. This causes physical deconditioning, which in turn results in more pain and so a vicious cycle is established. The increased steroid levels due to chronic stress response can, in addition, cause impairment in tissue growth and its repair and suppression of immunity.

Besides stress, physical deconditioning can happen due to changes in behaviour related to pain and activity avoidance. Noteworthy are the behavioural changes that cause restriction in normal physical activity, such as fear avoidance (fear of pain causing avoidance of activity), kinesiophobia (fear of movement) and pain catastrophizing.

Having explained how physical deconditioning contributes to chronic pain, I invited Dr Prakash to explain to the family the role of mental deconditioning in chronic pain. She explained that mental deconditioning is seen when distress natural to an illness or injury starts to take the form of fear. This gradually develops into psychological problems as seen by learned helplessness, anxiety-provoking thoughts, distorted thoughts (particularly catastrophizing thoughts), depression, personality changes and, perhaps even use, abuse and dependence on substances. These changes depend upon the pre-morbid personality and social environment of the person. Over a period of time, these emotional disturbances worsen and become chronic, thus leading to development of a sick role.

We could see Rahul had a thoughtful expression on his face as we approached the last chart.

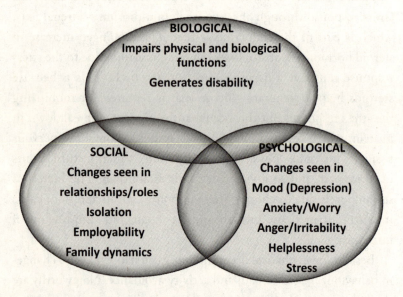

Fig 1.4: Chronic pain changes

Between Dr Prakash and I, we explained how chronic pain affects us physically, psychologically and socially. Repercussions of chronic pain are by far too many and too extensive to be ignored or side-lined as they play an important role in perpetuation of the pain experience. Physical pain affects activities of daily living such as walks, exercise and performing household chores. Besides, as we pointed out, in his case, it even prevented him from the simple pleasure of holding his child and playing with him. Physical pain can adversely impact physiological activities like sleep, bowel habits and appetite. Disability is another important repercussion of chronic pain. Disability is not just physical limitations such as standing, walking and performing household tasks, but includes limitation to perform self-care activities, ability to concentrate, ability to interact and socialize with people and carry on with one's occupation.

Psychological changes seen in chronic pain include fearfulness, worry, anxiety, helplessness, hopelessness, irritability, depression and stress related to coping with day-to-day living. Socially and economically, there is fear of dependency, fear of losing one's job, financial difficulties, family upheaval and distress and even change in social roles.

We both explained to Rahul that since chronic pain is multi-dimensional, its management, too, needs to be focused on dealing with all these aspects in toto, and not just the physical aspect. Hence, we should follow the multidisciplinary approach that would include, in his case, a pain specialist, orthopaedic specialist, clinical psychologist and physiotherapist. We assured him that as per our protocol, all of us customarily exchange notes for charting out an individualized multimodal and multidisciplinary treatment programme, so that all aspects of pain would be addressed simultaneously and each one of us is in the loop. Later on, we have review meetings to assess the patient's progress and to discuss further inputs that were still required to be incorporated.

Rahul looked at both of us and nodded. He said, 'I think I will come regularly for treatment, both physical and psychological. I recognize some of these issues are present in me too and these need to be addressed.'

We then explained to him that, in his case, he had chronic pain that was currently myofascial in origin secondary to the injuries that he had sustained. That besides the physical pain, he had other issues—psychological and social—that were contributing to his pain experience. This included depression and anxiety related to further pain and injury, inability to demonstrate his love for his child, guilt feelings related to the tragic fate of his friends, inability to manage himself, increase in irritability, role reversal, angst of family members and strained relationship with his spouse. He was even suffering from spiritual pain since he thought he was paying the penance for his past misdeeds and misadventures. All these aspects were adding to his pain experience.

He said, 'I think that instead of feeling sorry for myself, I need to get on with my life and take the necessary steps to do so. Let me start right here with you folks.' He smiled whimsically and added, 'What a dreadful way to grow up. I think I owe it to my son as well as Ravi's daughter to recover as much as possible. At least for my friend's sake, I can be a father figure to her.'

We too smiled back at him and pointed at Buddha's quote on the wall that read:

> The secret of health for both mind and body is not to mourn for the past, worry about the future, or anticipate troubles, but to live in the present moment wisely and earnestly.

Rahul concluded by saying, 'So I can safely say that to get better, I need to work both on my mind and body.' We both nodded and added, 'Yes, to manage your chronic pain.'

2

Decoding Chronic Pain

Pain is like a shadow that dogs our footsteps right from our birthing process, when the mother experiences severe pain, till the culmination of our life. Pain is a universal and ubiquitous phenomenon with far-reaching consequences not only in our physical body but in our psyche as well. The word pain is derived from the Latin word 'poena', which means penalty or punishment. 'Poine' in Greek also means payment or penalty, while the Anglo-French meaning of 'peine' is pain and suffering. But it must be noted that certain types of pain are protective in nature and are necessary for our safety and survival. The transition from protective functions, as seen in acute pain, to becoming chronic, debilitating and a disease is a worthy enough reason to differentiate between the types of pain.

Defining Pain

Pain, as mentioned earlier, is an unpleasant physical and emotional experience. For decades the concept of pain revolved around nociception ('nocere': to harm or hurt and 'ceptor': for receptor or sensor), which is the neural encoding of injury by the body. In other words, the unpleasant sensation caused by physical injury and tissue damage is conveyed by specific neurons to the brain where it is perceived as pain. In 1979, the International Association for the Study of Pain (IASP) defined pain as an 'unpleasant sensory and emotional experience associated with actual or potential tissue damage or described in terms of such damage.' It specifically mentions tissue damage for pain to be experienced. This definition has been subjected to various criticisms over the years based on patient experiences as well as on the improved understanding of pain. Advances in imaging technology and emerging research in the fields of pain medicine and mental health has provided us with a wealth of information and the realization that pain is not centred purely on nociception and tissue damage, but it can occur even without actual physical injury. Put simply, this means that nociception and pain are not synonymous with each other and pain can occur even without actual physical injury. Thus, there was a need to modify and update the definition of pain.

In July 2020, the IASP updated its forty-year-old definition of pain.[1] This was done by a task force and with inputs from multiple stakeholders including clinicians, researchers, philosophers and public, which included patients as well as their caregivers. The current definition of pain is: 'An unpleasant physical and emotional experience associated with, or resembling that associated with, actual or potential tissue damage.' The word 'resembling' implies that actual or even potential tissue damage need not necessarily be present for pain to occur. This definition provides the following updated notes to further clarify it:

- Pain is always a personal experience that is influenced to varying degrees by biological, social and psychological factors, which simply means that it is a biopsychosocial experience.

- Pain and nociception (sensing of physical injury) are different phenomena. Pain cannot be inferred solely on the activity of sensory neurons.
- Through their life experiences, individuals learn the concept of pain.
- A person's report of an experience as pain should be respected.
- Although pain usually serves as an adaptive role, it may have adverse effects on function and social and psychological well-being.
- Verbal description of pain is only one of several behaviours to express pain; inability to communicate does not negate the possibility that a human or a non-human/animal experiences pain.

This updated definition of pain along with the accompanying notes have clarified that pain is influenced by the interplay of multiple factors. Since these factors, which include psychological and social ones, tend to either heighten or diminish the pain, pain is more of a biopsychosocial experience. This has been a known fact since the late 1970s, when Engel,[2] a psychiatrist, proposed the 'biopsychosocial' model to explain any illness that also included pain. Meanwhile, Dame Cicely Saunders,[3] the pioneer of palliative care, had also embraced a more or less similar concept in her 'total pain' model, in which she described physical pain along with psychological, social and spiritual pain. In 1968, Margo McCafferty[4] had also stressed that, 'Pain is whatever the experiencing persons says it is existing, whenever he/she says it does.' Thus, many of the updated notes of the new definition of pain had already been stressed upon by eminent clinicians and mental health professionals in the past.

As explained, the new definition specifies that pain can occur even in the absence of tissue damage or injury (nociception). Therefore, it would be inappropriate to assume that the person is faking pain or that it is 'all in his/her head', when there is no specific underlying cause, as seen in psychological pain. In fact, WHO's International Classification of Diseases (ICD) 11th revision has for the first time given a classification of chronic pain and has acknowledged that tissue damage need not be necessarily present for chronic pain to occur. An added feature in the definition emphasizes that besides verbal self-report, while assessing pain one should also consider non-verbal expressions of the person. This is especially relevant in neonates, infants, those with intellectual disability and the elderly population, especially when their cognitive functions are declining or impaired (Alzheimer's disease or other types of dementias).

Lastly, the updates in the new definition mention that individuals learn pain through their life experiences. Since chronic pain brings much recompense if it is maintained, it often results in the development of a 'sick role'. In consequence, those activities that are adaptive and self-sustaining get extinguished as they do not bring adequate compensations.

Acute Pain, Chronic Pain and Chronic Pain Syndrome

Pain that is physiological is called acute pain. Usually, any pain starts off as acute pain; but when it persists for over twelve weeks it is termed as chronic pain. In chronic pain, physical pain alone does not define it as other perhaps more dominant, psychological and social factors compound it. Some of these psychosocial problems could be poor sleep, reduced performance at work, loss of job or loss of status in the family and society. All these factors are potentially stress inducing. When the person is unable to cope, it leads to stress, nervousness, anxiety and often depression. Since the pain pathways and the limbic system in the brain are functionally connected and activated together, any changes in the mood state trigger the nervous system. As pain is also a nerve-related phenomenon, the activated neurons cause an increase in the the perception of pain. This forms a vicious cycle as chronic pain begets psychosocial difficulties and they, in turn, beget more pain. Hence, when the psychological symptoms overshadow the physical symptoms, it is called chronic pain syndrome. To rephrase it, the mind starts to dominate over the body. In such patients, it is important to address the mind as much as we address the body, in order to relieve the suffering. And for that, a multidisciplinary approach of management is often required. In contrast to acute pain, pain in patients with chronic pain and chronic pain syndrome can become a double-edged sword when pain no longer has an adaptive and protective function but it, instead, becomes a *disease in itself* that causes disability and long-lasting suffering.

Acute Pain

Let us now try and understand the pain that is useful and protective (acute pain) and then see how pain ceases to be protective and instead becomes a disease (chronic pain).

As mentioned earlier, acute or physiological pain has both an adaptive and a protective function. While the adaptive function enables us to react appropriately to a threatening environment, the protective function warns of some impending tissue damage, injury or disease. In fact, this type of pain is needed for our very survival. It is termed physiological ('physio' means nature or natural) because it is normal to have this kind of pain and, in fact, not having it can be abnormal and even harmful. Congenital insensitivity to pain is a genetic disorder, which means a person is born with the inability to perceive physical pain and the absence of this protective sensation can adversely affect the lifespan of these individuals. This is because pain not only induces a reflex withdrawal from the injurious stimulus, but also initiates certain behavioural strategies that protect a person from further injury. An example would be withdrawal of the hand (reflex behaviour) when it is too close to fire (injurious stimulus). Thus, it is natural or physiological to experience pain after an injury, inflammation or surgery. There is also a stress response associated with acute pain depending on its severity, which is the fright, fight and flight response. This is termed as the autonomic response and it manifests as sweating, fast pulse rate, rapid breathing, raised blood pressure and dilatation of the pupils.

Acute pain lasts for only a short duration or till such time as the injury or tissue damage is present. It can affect our musculoskeletal system (somatic pain) or it can affect our internal organs or viscera (visceral pain). Some examples of acute pain are sprains, fractures, burns, surgery, cancer, arthritis or due to inflammation of internal organs like appendix, gall bladder or the urinary system, as in renal stones. Healing or resolution of the problem usually results in the pain abating and this time period is usually less than six weeks or a maximum of twelve weeks.

Chronic Pain

Now, let us see what happens in chronic pain. Pain is considered chronic when it has lasted for more than twelve weeks, persisting long after the healing period of an injury or inflammation is over. Although initially it might have had a beneficial function, but when it persists, it becomes a disease in itself causing distress and suffering and, hence, is termed as pathological pain ('pathos' means suffering). It has also been termed as dysfunctional pain as it serves no beneficial function, but rather causes impairment in functionality of the person and adversely affects the quality of life. Psychologically speaking, chronic pain is a major stressor to the patient and consequently to the family, as there may be fears related to uncertainty of regaining adequate functionality. The fear of dependency at all levels—physical, psychological and financial—may be present as an unwelcome appendage.

The same conditions that caused physiological pain can lead to or progress to pathological pain or chronic pain, except that while acute pain is largely due to tissue damage (nociceptive), in chronic pain multiple factors could be contributory and tissue injury may not always be present. In fact, in some cases of chronic pain, there may not be any underlying physical abnormality at all.

In contrast to acute pain, chronic pain tends to be more resistant to treatment. The prevalence of chronic pain worldwide is 20 per cent and is a cause of distress, disability and economic burden.[5] It is indeed heartening that for the first time in 2019, the classification of chronic pain has been included in WHO's ICD-11.[6] According to this classification there are seven groups of chronic pain, which broadly come under two major categories. These are as follows:

- Chronic primary pain
- Chronic secondary pain
    o Chronic cancer pain
    o Chronic post-traumatic or post-surgical pain
    o Chronic neuropathic pain
    o Chronic headache and orofacial pain
    o Chronic visceral pain
    o Chronic musculoskeletal pain

In chronic primary pain there is no other primary disease or disorder that could possibly contribute to the pain. This category includes psychological pain and widespread pain, as in fibromyalgia. Chronic secondary pain, on the other hand, is due to an underlying disease or conditions such as cancer, trauma or surgery, dysfunction of the nervous system, headaches and facial pains, musculoskeletal disorders or diseases in the organs of the body (visceral pain). These are discussed in greater detail in chapter four.

Chronic Pain Syndrome

Chronic pain syndrome is a little different from chronic pain and was delineated as a separate entity only in 1987. While in chronic pain, pain is the predominant symptom, in chronic pain syndrome, psychological symptoms are more prominent as compared to the physical symptoms of pain. Pain must be present for at least six months for it to be diagnosed as chronic pain syndrome. This condition is seen in approximately 25 per cent of patients with chronic pain. The psychological symptoms include depression, anxiety and mood-related changes such as lack of sleep, anger, frustration, loss of sexual desire, fatigue, irritability, guilt, substance abuse, marriage and family problems, job loss and even suicidal ideation. These symptoms become inextricably intertwined with pain and, in fact, become more dominant. So, what began as a simple tissue injury, gets affected by various physical, genetic, environmental and psychological factors—spiralling into a chronic pain condition where the psychological and social ramifications overshadow the physical symptoms.

Some of the common chronic pain conditions that lead to chronic pain syndrome are musculoskeletal disorders like various types of arthritis; neurological disorders like neuralgias (trigeminal, post-herpetic), migraine, cervical disc disease, degenerative spine disease; urological disorders like interstitial cystitis (inflammation of the urinary bladder), reproductive tract disease (endometriosis) and fibromyalgia. Other conditions such as treatment of cancer and chronic post-surgical pain are also perpetrators of chronic pain syndrome.

Psychological disorders that may make the person prone to develop chronic pain syndrome include major depression, dysthymia, anxiety disorders, some personality disorders and somatization disorders.

Understanding Chronic Pain

Briefly put, certain fundamental changes occur in the central nervous system that contribute to the chronicity of pain. The underlying cause of chronic pain is very complex. Despite advances in imaging technology and unending research in pain medicine, it is still not well understood. Suffice to say, besides the nervous system that is diseased, the muscles, the body's stress axis, the immune system, the mind and a host of other factors are also major contributors for the chronicity of pain.

To understand the mechanism of chronic pain better, we need to first have a clear understanding of the mechanism of acute or physiological pain. Although the classical pathway of pain was first described by Descartes[7] in the seventeenth century (Cartesian model), it is a subject of active research and is still evolving. He described four stages in the pain pathway: transduction, transmission, modulation and perception. The signal that is sensed in the periphery (transduction), after being transmitted and modulated, is ultimately perceived in the brain (Fig 2.1).

Nowadays, there is a trend to move away from the Cartesian model of the pathway of pain because nociception and tissue injury, which are considered transduction or the first stage of the pathway, are not always necessary for pain to be experienced. Nevertheless, we are mentioning this pathway in the context of understanding pain, as it is a simplistic way to understand how pain is ultimately perceived.

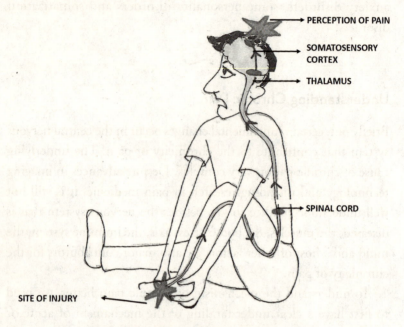

Fig 2.1: Pain pathway: The Cartesian model

How Do We Perceive Physiological Pain?

Whenever there is tissue damage or injury, a wide range of inflammatory mediators are released not only locally from damaged tissues but also by circulating blood cells at the injured site. These inflammatory mediators (bradykinin, prostaglandins, H^+, Na^+, K^+, histamine, serotonin, substance P, etc.) stimulate specialized sensors called nociceptors to detect pain. Nociceptors are present everywhere in our body—not only in the skin but also in the muscles, joints and various organs of the body. It can be specific for mechanical stimuli (mechanoceptor), thermal stimuli (thermal receptor), chemical receptors or it could be common for a wide range of mechanical, thermal and chemical stimuli (polymodal nociceptor). Some of these polymodal nociceptors can be silent or sleeping and are activated only when the injurious stimulus is sustained and prolonged or when there is associated inflammation as usually happens in chronic pain.

The pain stimulus sensed by the nociceptor is converted or transduced to an electrical impulse for it to be transmitted by nerves to the spinal cord and brain. This is the first stage of the pain pathway or transduction. The electrical stimulus is then transmitted through specific pain transmitting neurons (A delta and C fibres) to the spinal cord. The A delta nerves are thicker and have a covering of myelin (myelin sheath) that makes them conduct the pain impulse faster than the C fibres, which do not have a myelin sheath and are thinner as compared to the A delta nerves. Due to its faster conduction rate, the A delta transmits the 'first pain' signal, which is pricking and sharp and is felt soon after the injury, whereas the C fibres transmits 'second pain', which is the burning, dull and throbbing pain that is felt a few seconds later. Thus, transmission of the pain signal is the second stage of the pain pathway.

The sensation of touch is transmitted by the A beta nerve fibres, which have even thicker myelin sheath than the A delta nerve fibres and are also thicker in comparison to the ones that transmit pain. As a result, touch is transmitted much faster than pain. We are mentioning this because the mode of transmission of touch sensation has immense relevance in some types of chronic pain and in the Gate Control Theory of Pain, which will be elaborated upon later on.

The pain signal that is converted into an electrical impulse in the periphery (transduction) and gets transmitted through specific nerve fibres (transmission) now reaches the spinal cord. The spinal cord is not a passive structure meant only as a relay station for further transmission of pain to the brain, but plays a very crucial role in modulating the pain impulse by either diminishing or enhancing it. Let us see how.

In the spinal cord, the peripheral or first order neurons connect with the second order neurons (projection neurons). Besides, the first order neurons connect with shorter neurons called interneurons. The role of the interneurons is modulating the pain impulse by gating and prioritizing the incoming inputs within the confines of the spinal cord. The second order neurons or projection neurons, on the other hand, are much longer and are responsible for transmitting this modulated pain impulse to higher areas in the brain through ascending nerve tracts (Fig 2.2).

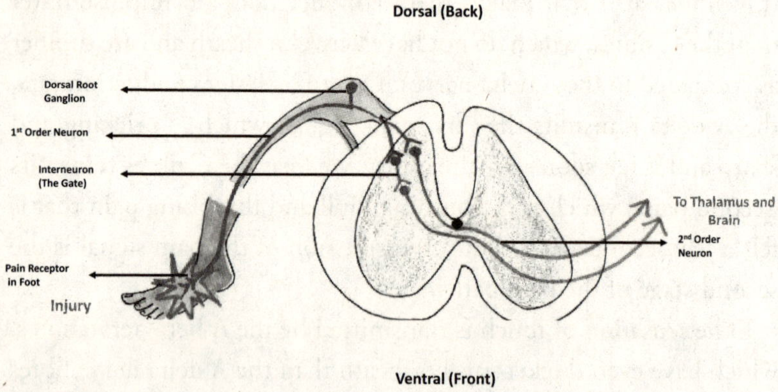

Fig 2.2: The pain pathway depicting the spinal cord with the first and second neurons and the dorsal root ganglion

The junctions between the neurons (synapse) are bridged by amino-acid-like substances called neurotransmitters, which transfer the information between the neurons. Based on the type of neurotransmitter that is released, the interneurons in the spinal cord modulate the incoming pain signal by either amplifying it (excitatory) or decreasing it (inhibitory). The excitatory interneurons release the excitatory neurotransmitter called glutamate and substance P; while the inhibitory interneurons release GABA, which is an inhibitory neurotransmitter that decreases the pain sensation.

The projection neuron or the second order neuron, which interfaces with the first order neuron, transmits the pain signal to the next station, the thalamus, which is situated in the depths of the brain. The thalamus is a major relay station for the pain impulse where the next junction (synapse) is present between the second and third order neuron. Thereafter, the third order neuron transmits the pain signal to multiple areas in the brain where the sensation of pain is perceived or experienced in its totality (stage of perception) (Fig 2.3).

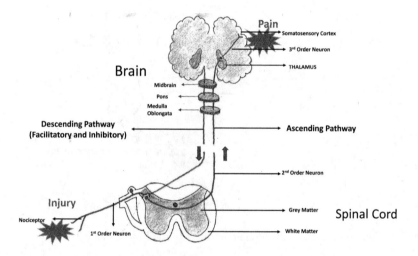

Fig 2.3: The pain pathway depicting the first, second and third order neuron, the dorsal root ganglion and the ascending and descending pathways

These centres in the brain constitute the somatosensory cortex (for localization and determining the intensity of pain), limbic area (for the emotional and motivational aspect of pain), prefrontal cortex (for the evaluative aspect of pain) and the motor area that determines the action that needs to be taken in response to the pain. The hypothalamus, which is situated in the base of the brain, is responsible for the stress response seen in pain and it stimulates the endocrine glands to release stress hormones. The areas concerned for sleep that includes the pineal gland are also affected by the pain stimulus.

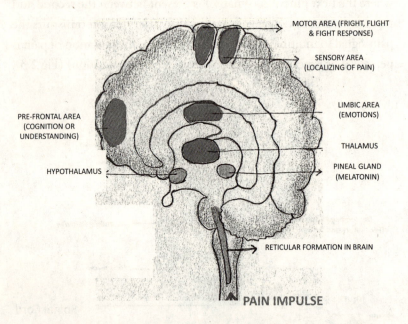

Fig 2.4: Projection of the pain impulse to multiple areas in the brain

Neuroimaging studies have confirmed that multiple areas of the brain are involved in processing the sensation of pain. This has been termed as the pain matrix. The pain experience is, thus, not just physical discrimination of pain as most of us think it is but has a motivational or affective aspect that involves our emotions, an evaluative aspect that includes our thoughts and actions and even elicits an autonomic response of the body to pain. The pain matrix explains how a person with a limb fracture experiences not only physical pain but has anxiety and fear (emotional reaction) along with palpitations and sweating (autonomic reactions). The evaluative aspect of the pain response that involves our thought processes ensures that the person is cognizant of the enormity of the situation and undertakes suitable steps to prevent further harm and take necessary action.

Meanwhile, en route to the brain, the ascending pain signal is relayed to subcortical areas of the brain (brain stem), which is just below the brain. From there, descending signals are sent down to the spinal cord that either amplify or decrease the pain signal (Fig 2.3). These are the descending excitatory or inhibitory pathways respectively that serve to modulate the original pain impulse. The descending inhibitory pathways decrease the pain sensation through the inhibitory neurotransmitters, namely serotonin and norepinephrine. In fact, many of the medications used to treat pain act by increasing these chemicals in our body.

Thus, we see that our body is equipped with an inbuilt analgesic system mediated by the inhibitory interneurons in the spinal cord (interneurons) and the descending inhibitory pathways from the brain. This inbuilt analgesic system includes the endogenous opioids like endorphins (as opposed to exogenously administered morphine), which helps to mitigate the pain response. Besides, our thoughts and emotions can play a major role in modulating the pain impulse.

A major boost to the understanding of the pain pathway came in 1965 with the Gate Control Theory of Pain proposed by Ronald Melzack and Patrick Wall.[8] They proposed that not all the pain impulses that come from the periphery are relayed to the brain and that there is a gating mechanism at the level of the spinal cord where these impulses are regulated, either inhibited or facilitated. These 'neural gates' are the path through which all sensory stimuli such as touch, pressure and pain are transmitted on their onward journey to the brain for perception. If non-painful stimuli like touch and pressure overpower the pain stimuli, it can close the gate for the pain stimuli, which are then not allowed to pass through and the perception of pain reduces. On the other hand, if the pain stimuli are in excess, the gate remains open for it to pass through and the pain is felt.

This is the mechanism by which massage, application of analgesic gels or even modalities used in physiotherapy such as TENS (Transcutaneous electrical nerve stimulation) and IFT (Interferential current) works. It is even one of the mechanisms by which acupuncture is proposed to work. These neural gates are also influenced by descending influences from the brain such as thoughts, emotions and even the activity level of the person. For example, when a person is concentrating on a task, they are momentarily distracted and do not feel so much pain and that is the basis of distraction therapy. Thus, various cognitive (ruminating about pain) and emotional factors (anxiety or depression) can influence the gate by either opening or closing it and thereby altering the perception of pain. Even the activity level of the person influences the gate. Boredom or lack of physical activity can open the gate and enhance the experience of pain, while remaining active has the opposite effect.[9]

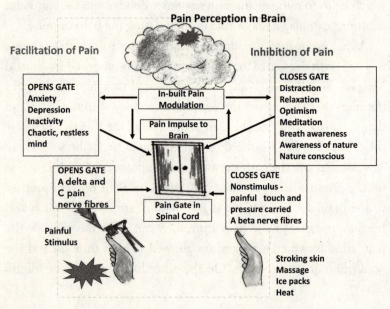

Fig 2.5: The Gate Control Theory of Pain

This is normal nociception and indicates what happens in acute or physiological pain.

What Happens in Chronic Pain?

Under certain conditions, pain can get transformed from being a temporary, protective phenomenon to a persistent, distressing 'disease'. This could happen when there is an ongoing tissue injury/inflammation that does not heal. Sometimes, when pain is severe and undertreated, it can transition into chronic pain as happened in the case of Rahul that was discussed in the first chapter. But it is not necessary that the transition from acute to chronic pain will happen only with severe injuries. Sometimes even a mild injurious stimulus can transform to chronic pain, as it happens in a condition called chronic regional pain syndrome. On the other hand, in neuralgia such as post-herpetic neuralgia or neurological illnesses like brain stroke, multiple sclerosis or spinal cord injury, it could be a disease or lesion in the nervous system that causes chronic pain. Finally, in central sensitization syndromes and psychogenic pain, there is no pathology that can account for the pain. It is basically due to an oversensitive central nervous system. In psychogenic pain, a significant psychological reason needs to be present to develop pain that then becomes an expression of distress, which is communicated in the form of physical pain. This kind of psychic pain is seen in psychological disorders like bodily distress disorder (previously termed as somatoform disorders), conversion reaction, depression and anxiety (autonomic symptoms). So, chronic pain can occur due to a number of reasons—some due to injury to various tissues and some where there is no injury whatsoever.

We have seen the sequence of events involved in the perception of acute pain; let us now see what happens in chronic pain. The events can be broadly categorized as: (a) changes at the site of injury;

(b) changes in the spinal cord; (c) changes in the brain; (d) the influence of ascending and descending pathways between the spinal cord and the brain.

Changes at the Site of Injury

When the injurious stimulus is prolonged and persistent or when there is extensive tissue injury or tissue damage as happens in cases of severe trauma/accidents or cancer, the tissue damage itself stimulates a prolonged inflammatory response. This is distinct from the transient inflammatory response seen in acute pain. In extensive trauma or chronic inflammation, a host of chemical pro-inflammatory mediators (prostaglandins, histamine and bradykinin) are released at the site of injury, akin to an 'inflammatory soup' that bathe the pain sensory neuron in it (Fig 2.4). This reaction, termed as peripheral sensitization, lowers the threshold to pain and results in an augmented response of the sensory fibres to pain. As a result, there is an increase in the amplitude of the pain response, which heightens the pain experience.

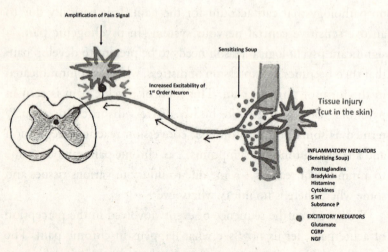

Fig 2.6: Peripheral sensitization

We had earlier alluded to silent nociceptors, which normally lie quiescent in acute pain. These get activated when there is prolonged inflammation. As a result, even innocuous stimuli that normally would not cause pain, become painful. For example, our joints have many receptors that can sense pain: the mechanoreceptors (specific for mechanical stimuli), polymodal receptors (common for mechanical, thermal and chemical stimuli) and silent nociceptors. In osteoarthritis of the knee, the inflammation in the joint activates the silent nociceptors, which start neuronal firing spontaneously even without movement and that contributes to the pain even at rest. On the other hand, the mechanoreceptors present in the joint get activated and cause pain while walking due to the mechanical pressure on these receptors when the person is in the upright position.

So, we can see that the main changes that occur in the periphery or at the site of injury is peripheral sensitization by pro-inflammatory chemicals and activation of silent nociceptors. These factors increase the sensitivity to pain and culminate in chronic pain, which is prolonged and out of proportion to the initial injury and, therefore, more distressing.

Changes in the Spinal Cord and Central Sensitization

The spinal cord has a major role to play in the chronicity of pain. The seat of activity is in the dorsal root ganglion and the dorsal horn of the spinal cord, which is situated in the rear part of the spinal cord all along the length of the spinal cord (Fig 2.2). The increased firing of the neurons from the site of injury as a result of peripheral sensitization, in turn, leads to sensitization of the neurons in the spinal cord with consequently an increased release of excitatory neurotransmitters. This further enhances the pain sensation—a phenomenon called central sensitization.

Besides, there is also activation of certain receptors in the spinal cord that adds to the chronicity of pain. One such receptor is the

NMDA receptor, which is not normally activated in acute pain, but gets activated when there is continuous and ongoing onslaught of pain stimuli from the periphery. This causes the spinal cord to undergo a 'wind up' akin to the volume of a radio, which blares loudly even though the volume control is at a minimum (Fig 2.7). As a result, the spinal cord becomes supersensitive to all kinds of incoming stimuli including non-painful ones like a simple touch. It simply means that besides responding to neurons that convey pain sensation (A delta and C neurons), the neurons in the dorsal horn of the spinal cord become supersensitive and respond even to A beta neurons that convey non-painful stimuli like touch. The dorsal horn of the spinal cord is also the site of the neural gates, which can increase or decrease the onward transmission of pain stimuli (see Gate Control Theory of Pain mentioned earlier).

Thus, we see that the spinal cord is not just a passive relay station for the pain impulse to traverse on its way to the brain, but it can actively increase or decrease the pain experience in various ways.

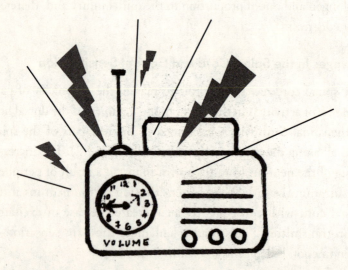

Fig 2.7: Central sensitization: radio blaring loudly even though volume is at minimum

To reiterate, the chain of events that start from peripheral sensitization, increased neuronal firing, activation of the NMDA receptor and 'wind up', ultimately leads to central sensitization, which is the hallmark of chronic pain and is contributory to the heightened pain response in chronic pain conditions.

The Brain and Central Sensitization

The constant bombardment of painful stimuli on the brain from below can cause its remodelling. This is termed as neuroplasticity. Simply put, neuroplasticity is the ability of the brain to change its structure and function depending on the circumstances. Normally, neuroplasticity is a positive adaption to a given situation, but in the case of chronic pain, it is maladaptive as it leads to the perpetuation of pain. The fact that the brain and spinal cord are very much responsible for chronic pain occurrence has been shown by neuroimaging studies, which have helped unravel, to a large extent, the processing of pain by the brain. This has been mostly studied in chronic pain conditions with central sensitization such as fibromyalgia, chronic low back pain, neuropathic pain and temporo-mandibular joint disease. In these patients, neuroimaging of the brain has shown structural changes in the pain processing areas. Besides change in structure, neurochemical alterations like increase in excitatory neurotransmitters and decrease in inhibitory transmitters has also been demonstrated. An increase in the resting brain network connectivity in areas of the brain that subserve pain and decrease in those areas that prevent pain has even been found in chronic pain conditions.

These findings suggest that chronic pain is due to tangible and proven changes occurring in the body and it is rather unworthy to say that, *'It is all in the head.'* Most patients would rather hear that chronicity of their pain is linked to actual physical causes for the fear of hearing the above statement. Nonetheless, psychological factors have an equal and, at times, a more important role in maintaining chronic pain. This does not necessarily cast aspersions on the patient, for after all, they are not faking the pain. It would be more prudent to say that occurrence of both physical and psychological trauma impact the body and psyche of a once healthy body and mind, and can trigger chronic pain conditions. Some instances of physical trauma could be stress due to a surgery, prolonged illness or previous hospitalization. Some of the psychological stressors could be associated with a troubled or failed relationship, post depression, sexual or physical abuse in childhood.

In the case of fibromyalgia, which is a central sensitization disorder, patients invariably give a history of either a physical insult or psychological trauma. A patient told us that she went through tremendous stress when she was the caregiver for her husband, who was bedridden for a couple of years. Another gave a history of severe postpartum depression following the delivery of her child many years ago. Yet another had a physical insult in the past due to a nose fracture while playing badminton, which required several hospitalizations and surgeries to set it right. A young lady with fibromyalgia in her early thirties gave the history of a broken relationship, which had affected her deeply. These are but some instances of how trauma, physical or psychological, can impact the body and mind, leading to the genesis of central sensitization disorders.

Psychological factors along with physical, environmental and social factors can foster the chronicity of pain by creating a state of increased reactivity of the nervous system. Once again, let us allude to the example of fibromyalgia. A patient reported of being constantly taunted by her father for complaining of pain all the time. She was stressed, humiliated and felt that her pain was not understood by the very people who brought her into this world. In another instance, a medical practitioner who worked as a resident doctor in a premier institution was continuously feeling that she could not keep up with the high standards of the hospital and this became a regular source of stress. Yet another went through a traumatic divorce. All these patients had, in common, high anxiety, fear-avoidance, depression and daily stressors that they found difficult to cope with. It is quite possible that in fibromyalgia the increased reactivity of the nervous system due to these stress factors led to perpetuation of widespread pain and other distressing symptoms such as sleep disturbance, fatigue and depression.

Changes in Modulation of Pain in Chronic Pain State

Having discussed the changes that occur at the site of injury, in the spinal cord and the brain, let us now see how modulation of pain is affected in chronic pain conditions. Modulation of pain is mainly subserved by the nerve pathways that ascend to the brain from the spinal cord and those that descend from the brain to the spinal cord. In patients with chronic pain, the interneurons at the spinal cord level are responsible for a loss of pain filtering mechanism and an increase in the excitatory neurotransmitters. As a result, there is facilitation of the pain impulse that leads to more pain being experienced. Besides, the nerve pathways going back and forth between the spinal cord and brain are also affected as seen in the increase in activity of the excitatory pathways that subserve pain and a suppression of the inhibitory pathways that decrease pain (Fig 2.3). Thus, the inbuilt analgesic system of our body goes awry in chronic pain.

Since central sensitization is one of the hallmarks of chronic pain, let us see how it is manifested. The two classical features of central sensitization, which are very often seen in patients with chronic pain, are allodynia and hyperalgesia.

Allodynia (in Greek, allos means other and odynia means pain) is the pain occurring with a non-painful stimulus like touch or stroking of the affected area. Besides touch, other non-painful stimuli such as breeze from a fan, brushing the hair or even washing that area can be painful. We had a patient with chronic regional pain syndrome of her arm, who would keep her arm covered with a cloth to prevent even a draught of air coming in contact with it, as she experienced pain if it did. Similarly, patients with migraine find brushing their hair painful as the scalp can become tender. Fibromyalgia is a classic example of allodynia where mere touching any part of the body causes pain.

Hyperalgesia (in Greek, hyper means over and algos means pain) is increased sensitivity to pain. In other words, the intensity of pain after a painful stimulus could be exaggerated and more prolonged than it should normally be. Sometimes the pain can extend even beyond the injured area (secondary hyperalgesia).

Besides pain and touch, other senses such as smell, sound and light are heightened and become increasingly painful in persons with central sensitization. For example, patients with migraine invariably complain of increased sensitivity to sound (phonophobia) and light (photophobia). These usually worsen their headache and they invariably prefer to be in a dark and quiet place. A patient who had glossopharyngeal neuralgia (irritation of the ninth cranial nerve causing pain in the tongue, tonsillar region, throat and ear), would often be unable to bear loud sounds like honking of cars as it would hurt her ear. Central sensitization had made her oversensitive to loud noises (phonophobia).

It is not just sensations that are heightened with central sensitization. Many other parts of the brain, which are part of the pain matrix, also get sensitized leading to cognitive, emotional and behavioural changes. Disturbances in cognitive functioning like poor attention span, attention fatigability, difficulty in concentration and short-term memory loss can occur. Emotional distress is heightened in these patients as seen by increased anxiety, nervousness, bouts of anger and irritability. Behavioural changes seen in central sensitization include erratic behaviour, poor consistency in following instructions, social withdrawal and a likelihood of development of sick role.

Initially, central sensitization may be reversible; but over a period of time, it can become irreversible especially when pain is long-lasting. The common conditions where central sensitization is seen are low back pain, chronic regional pain syndrome, chronic neck pain, chronic tension headaches, chronic migraine, rheumatoid arthritis, osteoarthritis of the knees, fibromyalgia, pelvic pain, temporomandibular disorders, irritable bowel syndrome, overactive bladder in women, chronic fatigue syndrome and neurological illnesses like stroke and spinal cord injury.

〜

After a glimpse of the chain of events leading to central sensitization, let us now see how and why it occurs. In neurological illnesses like stroke and spinal cord injury, it is quite plausible for central sensitization to occur as there is damage in the brain (stroke) or spinal cord (spinal cord injury), which could possibly affect the pain pathways in the central nervous system, disturb the normal processing of pain and cause the altered and heightened response to pain.

But how can sudden and recent onset low back pain or a cut in the finger transition into either chronic low back pain or chronic regional pain syndrome respectively? What happens in fibromyalgia, an example of central sensitization, where there is no tissue injury? In this condition, there is not only widespread pain all over the body but there is also associated depression, sleep disturbance, mental fogging, allergies and bowel disturbances. What about the gynaecological problem endometriosis, in which the lower abdomen pain due to dysmenorrhea becomes so incapacitating that the pain spreads to the whole pelvic region, perineum, back and even the legs? Why do patients with migraine headaches have a sensitive scalp that even combing the hair becomes painful, besides making them oversensitive to non-painful stimuli like light and sound?

There are no clear answers to many of these questions. But there is a growing recognition that the underlying cause for this overlap of symptoms in the above-mentioned conditions is due to lowered threshold for perception of any sensory information, and not just the sensation of pain because of a highly strung central nervous system. It is noteworthy that in some chronic pain conditions like fibromyalgia, chronic headaches, temporomandibular joint disorders and pelvic pain, there is a significant overlap in symptoms. Persistent pain is a common denominator in these diseases, but other symptoms such as fatigue, sleep disturbance, bowel disturbances, dizziness, cognitive problems, depression and anxiety may be present in all of them to varying degrees. Hence, this group of disorders have been termed as central sensitization syndromes.

To summarize:
- Persistent or ongoing pain causes sensitization in the peripheral nerves conveying pain (peripheral sensitization), which leads to constant bombardment of the spinal cord neurons. This happens when there is ongoing inflammation, delay in the healing process or inadequately treated pain.
- Central sensitization, wherein the constant activation of the spinal cord neurons and brain by pain stimuli coming from the peripheral neurons causes them to undergo remodelling (neuroplasticity). They then become hypersensitive to even innocuous or trivial stimuli. Psychological, genetic and environmental factors can contribute to central sensitization.
- Abnormalities in the body's stress axis and disturbed hormonal regulation.
- Psychological causes such as learned behaviour, environmental and social factors play a major role in the occurrence of chronic pain. These will be discussed at length in the following chapter.

To conclude, the transition of pain from acute to chronic is still not understood well. It may involve multiple factors: physical, psychological and environmental. While acute or nociceptive pain is usually due to tissue injury and heals in a specified time frame, chronic pain may be due to a combination of both tissue injury and nerve damage with added muscle involvement. Chronic pain can even occur without any underlying physical cause. But the final common pathway is central sensitization and maladaptive changes in the spinal cord and brain, not to mention the psychological changes that take place in the individual.

3

Chronic Pain and the Mind: The Indivisible Phenomenon

'If your body is screaming in pain, whether the pain is muscular contractions, anxiety, depression, asthma or arthritis, a first step in releasing the pain may be making the connection between your body pain and the cause. Beliefs are physical. A thought held long enough and repeated enough becomes a belief. The belief then becomes biology.'

—Marilyn Van M. Derbur

These touching words make one pause and consider how chronic pain is related to the mind and the body. When a person has lived with pain for a long time, that pain becomes a part of their life. This constant onslaught of pain shapes their mental process and determines their emotional responses, which can range from anger and irritation to low mood, apprehension and apathy. This phenomenon had been documented from ancient times though not in explicit terms.

Ancient wisdom recognized that pain was universal, unavoidable and mostly sporadic, originating from physical injury. The source was external and believed to be inflicted by evil demons. Chronic pain, on the other hand, was not really understood except that its genesis was most likely related to the past sins that one may have committed. This bracketed pain more as a punishment for the misdeeds committed instead of being recognized as a physical and psychological event. Interestingly, since primordial times, pain as a feeling has been well-documented in all kinds of narrative forms. In Greek mythology, the Algea were personifications of pain, both physical and mental. They were related to Oizys, the Greek Goddess who represents the milder version of misery and sadness, and Penthos, the God of mourning and lamentation. The Greek word 'algos' is a neuter noun literally meaning pain and is used as a suffix for some painful conditions such as myalgia (muscle pain), neuralgia (nerve pain), arthralgia (joint pain) and so on. Through these fables, although ingrained but not explicit, one can infer that pain and emotions were seen as being related to each other.

Mind-Body dualism

Humans are the only species that have the unique ability for higher order thinking. This distinctive feature in mankind has led to much debate on how to define the nature of the relationship between the body and the mind, giving rise to the concept of dualism. Dualism denotes that the body and mind are two distinct entities. Gautama Buddha, who lived in the sixth or the fifth century BCE, described the mind and body as being co-dependent—like two sheaves of reed each leaning against the other and working interdependently in tandem. Much later, in the seventeenth century, Descartes postulated that the mind exerted control over the body through the pineal gland. This was called Cartesian dualism or substance dualism. He believed that though the mind was different from the body, it had the power to influence the body.

Although Descartes said that the 'soul' existed in the brain (pineal gland), later thinkers believed that this statement was made to escape religious persecution. However, this viewpoint, also referred to as the interactionism theory (Descartes, 1596–1650),[1] suggested that mind and body are two different entities and that they interact via the pineal gland, which is a tiny structure at the centre of the brain. He called this as the 'seat of the soul' since thoughts were supposed to be formed here. The body, in his opinion, had control over the rational mind and a two-way relationship existed between the mind and the body.

The interactionism theory was modified several times; its main proponents being Karl Popper, a science philosopher, and John Carew Eccles,[2] a neurophysiologist. The modified thinking gave rise to Emergentism.[3] This viewpoint asserts that mental states are the resultant of states of the brain and so the mental states can influence the brain, leading to a two-way communication between the mind and the body. In other words, the mind influences the body and vice versa.

Later, Epiphenomenalism[4] suggested that mental events in the brain could be caused by physical events, but these mental events may have no bearing on the physical events. The emotions we feel are caused by chemicals that interact with the body and are independent of the mind. Psychophysical parallelism[5,6] explains that body and mind are mutually exclusive of each other and although there is no communication between them, both react simultaneously. Double aspectism[7] went further and felt that both body and mind react concurrently but the phenomenon cannot be separated from each other. Two other schools, Pre-established Harmony[8] and Occasionalism,[9] also considered mind and body being distinct entities, but controlled by God.

Current Understanding of Mind-Body Phenomena

A breakthrough in understanding the mind-body phenomena pre-eminently came from cognitive psychologists. They compared the human brain to a computer's artificial intelligence. Just as the computer's hardware is wired, so is the brain connected to the body. Mind is like the software of the body that allows multiple and different reactions to the same stimulus. This rationale is in tandem with the cognitive mediational process. According to this process, our emotions are determined by our appraisal of the stimulus and our mental processes (memory, attention, perception and problem-solving abilities) act as mediation or go-between to produce a response.[10] Thus, mediation process occurs after the presentation of the stimulus but before the onset of the response. This was diametrically opposite to Descartes' view that stated, 'I think, therefore I am.'

Neuropsychologists and neuroscientists, using functional MRI, have physically verified that any reaction made by a person can be detected ten seconds in advance by scanning the brain activity. Hence, when a physical phenomenon like pain is felt, a neural network in the brain is simultaneously activated that produces the discriminative, cognitive, emotional and behavioural response to pain. This indicates that cognitive processes do have a physical basis in the brain as alluded to in the previous chapter.

Synthesizing of Thoughts, Emotions and Actions in Chronic Pain

According to psychologists, human beings are governed by their thoughts (cognitions) and emotions (affect), and together these direct the person's behaviour (conations). This combination of thought-emotion-behaviour has an invaluable function for human existence and survival. This is especially seen with acute pain where it has a survival value as it draws attention to the noxious stimulus and precipitates subsequent withdrawal response. In other words, perception of the noxious stimulus is processed in the brain, thoughts of danger are generated, then corresponding emotional response of fear and anxiety maybe felt, and the appropriate behavioural response of withdrawal from the noxious stimulus is activated.

Chronic pain experience, too, can be explained similarly. The thoughts and beliefs about pain (cognitions), creates fear, anxiety and depression (emotions) that, in turn, causes suffering. Thoughts and emotions eventually determine whether the person would be seeking active help or avoiding the situation (behaviour). Let us explain it in more detail.

Thoughts

Thoughts are influenced by the beliefs, attitudes and the cognitive set of the person. Beliefs are like timesavers that help the brain to process swiftly a large amount of incoming information (reaction to painful stimuli) for quick analysis. Since beliefs are a repertoire in the cognitive set of a person and are already ingrained in the mind, they provide a sort of automatic interpretation of the stimuli. In acute or sudden pain, they are instrumental in taking necessary and prompt action which, in turn, helps in adaptation to the situation. However, sometimes beliefs can have reverse reaction insofar as seeking treatment is concerned. If the belief system belies the benefits of certain type of treatment, then despite pain the person may actually refuse it. This is especially so in chronic pain where beliefs and attitudes can play a significant role. When the beliefs, attitudes, perception and treatment modalities are in consonance, a more positive approach for treatment is seen. The reverse is also true, and that contributes to chronicity of pain.

Another dimension to our cognitions is the cognitive set of a person. Cognitive set is the way we think. A rigid cognitive set prevents timely adaptation as the actual events can be misrepresented in the mind. This happens when cognitions get distorted as seen in catastrophic thinking. Catastrophic thoughts are exaggerated negative thoughts that tend to view even neutral situations as threatening. In the context of pain, catastrophic thoughts may interpret constant pain as indicative of serious underlying disease foreboding suffering and disability.

Emotions

When the thoughts are negative, pessimism is the automatic emotional response. Pessimism may relate well with other emotions of fear, anxiety, expressed and unexpressed anger, guilt, worry, depression, frustration and distress. Negative emotions increase the intensity of the pain experience, especially when worry is the chief component. It is interesting to note that one of the symptoms seen most often in depression is somatic or bodily complaints. Not only is pain experienced by a depressed person, but the intensity of already present pain increases sharply. Similarly, high anxiety, which generates autonomic symptoms (reactions of the body to anxiety), is also known to heighten the pain experienced. These are all suggestive of the fact that while dealing with chronic pain, emotions and emotional regulation need to be enforced.

Let us understand what is emotional regulation? It is the ability to exert control over one's own emotional state to be able to promote positive affect states. Emotions are markedly influenced by neurotransmitters released in the body such as dopamine, norepinephrine and serotonin. Serotonin is the most widely distributed neurotransmitter in the brain which is involved in emotional regulation particularly in depression, anxiety, stress response, impulsivity and aggression. Serotonin and dopamine are among the 'happy hormones' or 'feel-good' substances of our body. Some activities like physical exercises, laughter and meditation help release these neurotransmitters, which make a person feel cheerful and can ameliorate pain too.

Behaviour

Pain as a learned behaviour was a proposition put forth by Wilbert E. Fordyce[11] in the 1970s. He suggested that 'operant conditioning' was the key to understanding pain behaviour. Operant conditioning refers to the occurrence of behaviour that is brought about when something 'operates on the environment'. In other words, a person operates or manipulates the environment or performs some action that brings a reward. Learning of any behaviour is governed by this association of activity and reward.

Fordyce explained pain behaviour with the help of two tenets. The first tenet asserted that the behaviour that may have been beneficial for pain relief for short-term purposes could actually be potentially harmful in the long run. For instance, rest and analgesics may be required for short duration in the acute phase of pain but prolonged use of either or both may actually be detrimental, as exercise and muscle activity is the key to recovery in the long run. The second tenet spoke of learning of pain behaviour as being an interaction between the person and the social environment. Certain pain behaviours get reinforced due to the person's social and environmental milieu. For instance, if a person is exempted from certain activities and responsibilities due to pain, the avoidance of those tasks is the reinforcing agent. This is similar to secondary gains.

Chronic Pain and the Mind: Explaining the Indivisible Phenomenon

We have seen how thoughts, emotions and behaviour are interdependent on each other. In a similar fashion, the soma (body) and the mind are closely interlinked, with each having a significant impact on the other. While experiencing emotions like fear, anger or anxiety, we see the body reacting physically in a variety of ways.

One can either have a fight or flight response with an increase in heart rate, rapid breathing and tensing of muscles in preparation for action. However, when a person is feeling relaxed and contented, the exact opposite happens—the heart rate and breathing slows down and the muscles relax. Similarly, it has been found that chronic pain and many psychological disorders like depression, anxiety and stress, to name a few, coexist. Why do they tend to occur together? This can be explained based on the biopsychosocial model.

Let us consider the biological factors common to both chronic pain and the mind. Firstly, it has been found that deficiencies in the neurotransmitters, dopamine, serotonin and norepinephrine are common in both chronic pain conditions and certain psychological disorders. Depression is due to depletion of serotonin, dopamine and norepinephrine and is most strongly correlated with chronic pain. Antidepressants, which are commonly administered to patients with both depression and chronic pain, help to boost these substances in the body. Antidepressants serve a dual purpose of enhancing mood as well as relieving pain. Secondly, dysfunction of the body's stress mechanism, the hypothalamic-pituitary-adrenal axis, has been implicated both in chronic pain and mental disorders like anxiety, depression, substance abuse and post-traumatic stress disorder (PTSD). Lastly, functional MRI, which shows real-time activity in the brain, has revealed that in both chronic pain and mental disorders, certain common areas of the brain are involved. This further explains the link between them.

Likewise, certain psychological factors are also seen in common with chronic pain. These could include both mental processes and emotional state, which can alter the strength of pain perception. Mental processes could be attention span, self-control, comprehending the adversity of the situation and expectations of outcomes. Emotional mood state could be anxiety characterized by hypervigilance, catastrophizing, loss of control and autonomic symptoms. In depression, somatic complaints, hopelessness, helplessness, worthlessness and sleep disturbance are present. Common to both emotional mood state and chronic pain are catastrophizing thoughts and other distorted thoughts. Some personality types who can be more prone to chronic pain include the personality trait of neuroticism and two types of personality disorders: clusters B (Dramatic type) and C (Avoidant Fearful type). These will be discussed later on in the book.

Social aspects that influence pain cannot be overlooked. Adult chronic pain conditions can sometimes be traced to early childhood experiences. How pain is expressed or communicated in childhood and the response to pain by parents has a bearing on adult pain behaviour. Certain plausible reasons for pain behaviour in adult life include childhood interactions with parents, parents' solicitous reaction to pain and the child's strong and sympathetic identification with significant persons who have pain conditions. Interestingly, persons with persistent pain often have a history of physical and sexual abuse, especially in childhood. Such traumatized children grow up feeling inadequate, anxious and with somatic preoccupation. In fact, pain becomes an expression of distress from external threatening environment.[12] Chronic pain patients often find themselves being socially isolated, lonely, neglected, facing severe or long-term stress, having employability issues or being dissatisfied with their work. Family and marital dysfunctionality are concomitantly present. Sometimes chronic pain conditions become a source of righting the skewness within the family or a couple's relationship; at other times, it deteriorates an already strained situation.

Models Explaining the Mind-Body Interaction

Various models have tried to explain the indivisibility of mind and body and how, in chronic pain, the trinity of thoughts, emotions and behaviour supersedes the actual physical pain. Let us narrate two cases that were superficially similar, but which also illustrate how the body and mind are co-dependent in maintaining chronic pain. Both the patients were fifty-eight years old and living in joint families with their spouses, married sons, daughters-in-law and grandchildren. They belonged to affluent families and were homemakers. Each was a matriarch in her house and her word was law, which the rest of the family had to follow. But when we met the patients, we realized there were wheels within wheels and it took only a trivial incident to blow out of proportion and manifest pain, disability and suffering in them.

Mrs Annu had slipped on a ball left lying around carelessly by her granddaughter. She had not actually fallen but had only slipped and managed to steady herself by clutching the door. She had felt a jerk on her back (lumbar region) and had momentarily been unable to straighten her posture. Her first reaction was blinding rage at her daughter-in-law and granddaughter for leaving the ball lying around, when she had repeatedly reprimanded them for this laxity. In fact, she had always said in so many words that someday someone would get badly injured because of it. Her second reaction was the experience of sharp pain in her back. The same evening her pain worsened and despite applying analgesic gels, the pain did not subside leaving her sleepless, restless and extremely angry. Next day, her family consulted a doctor who advised her to apply cold packs, analgesics and take rest for a few days. Gradually, she improved and became almost pain-free.

Six weeks later, her daughter-in-law and granddaughter were again playing with the ball. The child suddenly expressed the urge to go to the washroom. Her mother hastily carried her away and so once again the ball was left lying around on the floor. While walking across the room the ball got entangled in Mrs Annu's clothes and almost made her trip and fall. The sudden jerk of a movement once again caused pain in her back, which had only just recovered from the previous episode. Once again, she felt anger amounting almost to a rage. She screamed so much in anger and pain that she felt dizzy and collapsed on the floor. Her screams brought the rest of the family running and seeing her condition, everyone reprimanded the daughter-in-law for her carelessness.

A second round of doctor visits started. This time, however, Mrs Annu did not get relief. Instead, she started becoming hypervigilant about not only objects left lying on the floor but also if anyone came near her, for fear of getting hurt again. The daily visits of her daughter and grandchildren were no longer a happy occasion as she would be apprehensive of getting injured whenever her grandchildren climbed on her lap or wanted to play with her. It made her angry and distressed and, in her mind, she blamed her daughter-in-law as being the cause of her discomfort. She had also expected to be cared for diligently by the perpetrator of her pain but that did not happen, and it irked her further.

After explaining the history to us, the family further elucidated that Mrs Annu was an emotionally volatile person, which induced the family to always maintain a respectful distance from her. Her husband added that ever since their marriage, seeing her volatility, he and his family had avoided any confrontations with her to maintain peace and harmony in the house. In fact, he often withdrew from arguments as any disagreement with her would bring on a hysterical reaction. Her children, two sons and a daughter, would also do their utmost not to be the cause of any of these emotional outbursts. The only person who openly defied her was her daughter-in-law, who neither followed her commands, nor appeared affected by her criticism. This was a source of persistent irritation to Mrs Annu.

After three years of unrelieved pain and reduced mobility, her family doctor referred her to our pain clinic. But seeing her overwhelmingly distressed, Dr Abraham decided to first send her for psychological evaluation.

The second patient was Mrs Soma, who also had a fall and developed low back pain because of it. When home remedies did not help, she sought medical treatment after a month of her fall. She was started on oral analgesics and referred for physiotherapy, which benefited her and helped subside the pain. But seven months later, the strap of her slipper snapped while she was in the bathroom and once again she fell on her back. Not only did her back pain recur, but now it radiated down her right leg. She was in considerable pain making it difficult for her to either stand or lie comfortably in bed. An MRI of her spine revealed disc protrusion at the lumbar level and she was advised bed rest, analgesics and physiotherapy. But the pain did not improve, instead, it tended to flare up each time she strained herself. Different specialists were consulted who reiterated that there was no need for any kind of surgical intervention and gave the same advice. Lying in bed became a norm for her as each time she would try moving around she would experience severe pain. Her family insisted that she continue the bed rest as they felt that her underlying condition had probably not yet healed. This went on for four years—and by this time Mrs Soma and her family believed that irreversible changes had taken place in her spine, which was perpetrating the chronic pain.

Suspecting that the lady was suffering from depression, one of her doctors referred her to Dr Prakash. On hearing her history, she suggested that before any psychological assessment or intervention was done, a fresh look at her back would be helpful. Initially, the family was reluctant to involve any more doctors because despite consulting so many, her pain had not improved. Their main concern was that a once happy-go-lucky and active person was now bedridden and depressed and had lost the will to help herself. She often spoke of death as the only way out of her misery and even had suicidal thoughts. As she was in a wheelchair, the hospital attendant first took her to our pain clinic.

Mrs Annu and Mrs Soma already had chronic pain when they were referred for psychological intervention. However, there was a marked difference in how both reacted to their pain.

Mrs Annu, when psychologically tested, showed significant anxiety for another fall. She was scared to exercise or walk around even in the house and carried anger, almost to the verge of rage, towards her daughter-in-law and granddaughter. The anger seemed to be stemming from the fact that her son had married against her wishes, and he had always stood by his wife. Mrs Annu was not even permitted to reprimand her. Her daughter-in-law willingly did the duties assigned to her in the house, but after that she usually busied herself with her child and mainly kept to herself. This rather infuriated Mrs Annu, as she felt slighted by her behaviour. She had indeed carried this impotent rage within her for years. Since she wanted her first grandchild to be a male, the granddaughter had further added to her grievance. As mentioned earlier, she held both her daughter-in-law and granddaughter responsible for her condition. In fact, it almost amounted to secondary gains (advantage that occur secondary to stated or real illness) by remaining in pain.

Mrs Soma's assessments, on the other hand, showed severe depression with suicidal ideation. She felt that remaining bedridden made her life worthless and useless. She felt neglected and uncared for as everyone was busy with their respective lives; no one was any longer spending time with her or taking care of her. Her family, however, refuted that, saying all of them had so arranged their work schedule that there was always a family member at home with her and even a dedicated housemaid had been employed for her alone. At that point, it was difficult to say whether Mrs Soma had depressive cognitions or, as often happens in chronic conditions, the family feels that they are doing enough but the sufferer still feels affronted and neglected.

Let us see how the various psychological models explain the link between the mind and chronic pain and extrapolate it to the above two cited cases.

Fear-avoidance Model

This model was conceptualized by Letham et al. (1983)[13] to explain why pain-related fears could cause chronic pain as a result of attentional processes and avoidant behaviour. The differences in thinking and emotions govern the development of chronic pain.

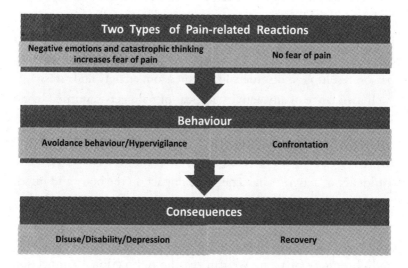

Fig 3.1: Fear-avoidance model

As the above diagram indicates, following an injury, distorted thought appraisals about the pain and the resultant negative feelings thus generated, leads to avoidance of activities of daily living (ADL) along with hypervigilance of bodily sensations. This continuous misrepresentation is characteristic of catastrophic thinking, which induces the individual to avoid any activity that has the potential of provoking pain. This eventually results in over-estimation of pain (Fig 3.1).

Fear-avoidance theory has emphasized that in chronic pain the emotional regulator, fear, is the key factor that perpetuates pain and causes the adverse sequelae of chronic pain. Fear develops as the thought associated with it—pain—is threatening (catastrophizing of thoughts) and, therefore, demands more attention (hypervigilance). That, in turn, leads to avoidance behaviour (inactivity or avoidance of activity) and ultimately to disuse, physical deconditioning, depression and disability. Disability then impacts the functionality of the person be it occupational, social, personal and recreational. Restrictions forced by disability have an adverse effect on the emotions of the person resulting in disorders like depression, anxiety and stress.

If avoidance of any activity for fear of pain gets rewarded by no increase in pain, then this behaviour gets positively reinforced. This may be beneficial in acute pain as restricted activities or rest helps in the healing process. However, in chronic pain, the fear of pain and avoidance of activities has a negative impact on the body and mind.

Thus, psychological factors such as fear of re-injury, dread of being in pain and avoidance of the activities that are perceived to increase pain enhances the likelihood of physical problems such as disability and chronicity of pain. We can see the bidirectional connection between the mind and the body. Physical pain leads to psychological problems, which, in turn, aggravate the physical condition.

In Mrs Annu's case, she was clearly fearful of re-injury and was hypervigilant about any fall, despite the fact that no actual injury had taken place. Her fears were not allowing her to relax and walk about freely in the house. Besides, she also carried so much of anger against her daughter-in-law and granddaughter that it added to the emotional component of pain. Since she felt helpless and powerless in venting out her anger, frustrations and fears, it actually made her depressed. Apart from feeling physical pain, she had become emotionally unwell too.

Now let us explore another psychological model that can further explain chronic pain.

Diathesis-stress Model

Stress is one of the most commonly used words in medical, psychological, social and cultural phraseology. Stress, a term which was first introduced and conceived by Hans Selye (1974)[14] in psychology, was simply described as the body's response to any physical, emotional or psychological strain. Subsequently, the term stress has been reframed as 'a particular relationship between the person and the environment that is appraised by the person as being taxing or exceeding his or her resources and endangering his or her well-being.'[15] Thus, psychological stress has been considered as an emotional strain and pressure that causes distress.

Stress has been categorized into two distinct types: daily hassles or chronic stress i.e., those that occur in our day-to-day life; and as life events or those that occur once in a lifetime. Both kinds of stress leave an impact on the human psyche. Due to its chronicity, daily hassles are more potent in debilitating a person's life. Despite the enormity and plethora of daily hassles, not everyone finds it difficult to cope with them as many have some innate capabilities to tide over them. However, some individuals may not be able to tackle so many difficulties and pressures. This could be explained by the presence of the 'vulnerability factor' that causes individual variation in appraising and responding to stress. Those who have proneness to stress would have low threshold to stress triggers and would succumb to it even with minor incidences. As a consequence, they could develop psychopathologies like depression, anxiety, distress or other psychological disorders.

Having understood what stress is, let us now understand the diathesis-stress model and the role it plays in the genesis and perpetuation of chronic pain.

The diathesis-stress model[16,17,18] tries to explain the development of chronic pain as a result of interaction between pre-dispositional vulnerability (diathesis) and stress (Fig 3.2). In other words, the diathesis or predisposition of the individual interacts with the person's stress resulting in chronic pain. This has been explained in the context of low back pain where the person's diathesis (pre-existing physical characteristics) interacts with intense and recurrent stressful factors (stress) and inadequate coping mechanisms ensuing in chronic low back pain.[19,20]

The stress model can be interpreted in another way, too. Chronic pain could be the stressor that activates the person's pre-existing psychological traits. The stress could either be physical pain itself or it could be due to the secondary losses (financial loss or disability) as a result of the pain.

To summarize, stress is any situation or series of situations or even life events that manage to disrupt the person's equilibrium. How the person, with his or her predisposition, perceives stress would, in turn, ascertain the reaction to the stress (stress response) and, subsequently, determine whether any disorder would develop. In other words, the model tries to explore how the genetic or biological predisposition or diathesis (say anxiety proneness) reacts to the stressful situation (say injury) for the person to develop any kind of disorder (say chronic pain).

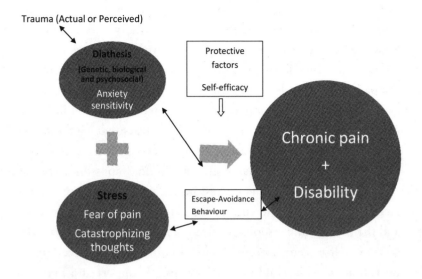

Fig 3.2: Schematic representation of diathesis-stress model

The predisposition or vulnerability of the person that make a person vulnerable to stress could be genetic, biological or psychosocial. The genetic factors usually remain restrained in a person till the person encounters a stressful situation. Biological factors include birth trauma, poor nutrition or deficiencies in early childhood. Psychological as well as social factors that include early childhood experiences of loneliness, maternal deprivation, social isolation, living in difficult and destitute conditions, sexual and physical abuse, extreme shyness, not having a sense of belongingness and anxiety sensitivity.

Anxiety sensitivity is a diathesis or a vulnerability factor that could play an important role in stress-induced chronic pain. Anxiety sensitivity literally means fear of sensations or behaviour that is induced due to anxiety. These sensations are misinterpreted by the individual as being harmful, dangerous and deleterious to their health. In chronic pain, high anxiety sensitivity makes a person hypervigilant to sensations that could cause pain, as seen in Mrs Annu's case. The selective attention that is paid to every sensation by the patient, in fact, leads to greater arousal, which tend to amplify even minor sensations and are then perceived as threatening. The perception of threat, in turn, enhances the fears that aggravate the avoidance behaviour (fear-avoidance). Over a period of time, this becomes a cyclical chain that is difficult but not impossible to break.

Between the diathesis and stress lie certain modifying protective factors that make a difference to the perception, thought processes and the behavioural response to stress. These attributes may be self-efficacy, self-esteem, internal locus of control, supportive family, nurturance during childhood, strong social support and network of friends, protective social environment and no history of prior physical or sexual abuse. These factors can have a beneficial effect on the person enabling them to cope with stress.

Of the above factors, self-efficacy has an important role to play in the perception of stress. Self-efficacy is the belief that a person carries about their innate ability to execute behaviour in order to produce a desired outcome.[21,22] In chronic pain, self-efficacy is considered as present when the belief to carry out certain activities is present in the sufferer, even when experiencing pain. It has an inverse relationship with predisposition to anxiety sensitivity. In other words, the lower the self-efficacy, the higher would be the anxiety sensitivity. A person with high self-efficacy would have a lesser tendency to be anxious and would be more confident to deal with a stressful situation.

Cognitive Processes in Chronic Pain

Cognitive (thinking) processes can often be extreme or catastrophic in patients with chronic pain. Catastrophic thinking is an irrational or distorted thinking process where the person ruminates about the worst-case scenario. In chronic pain, catastrophic thinking is seen in the beliefs the person has about the (a) cause and meaning of the symptoms, (b) anticipation of which symptom would cause what type and intensity of pain, (c) how much further damage is likely to happen to the body and (d) how the person would cope with the pain. Coping mechanism would depend on the degree of self-efficacy the person possesses. Thus, cognitions or thought processes have an effect not only on the physical and psychological functioning of the patient but could determine the compliance and outcome of the treatment process.

Some common cognition that one sees with chronic pain patients are as follows:

- Pain means that some damage has occurred to the body.
- Constant pain will lead to disability.
- Physical activity is harmful for my body so I should reduce them.
- Pain is permanent and very unlikely to decrease.
- There is no cure for chronic pain and one has to endure it lifelong.
- Movement worsens pain.
- Chronic pain is the result of my past deeds/sins.
- Chronic pain is a form of punishment.

And many such catastrophic and negative thoughts.

We saw in Mrs Soma's case that her depression was related to such catastrophizing thoughts. She had come to believe that any kind of physical activity or exercise would only increase her pain and so she continued taking bed rest. She even expressed anger at her family, saying she felt they already knew from doctors that she would never recover and were not revealing the reality of the situation to her. The negative thoughts related to pain had increased when the physiotherapist made her do some warm-up exercises and her pain increased. Since she had not exercised for more than a year, even minor movements were difficult for her to do. During the course of bed rest and inactivity, her muscles had become very weak and it required monumental efforts to persuade her to restart her physical therapy as she could barely stand or walk. It was evident right from the beginning that to help her one had to first work with her mind and then her body.

Acceptance and Commitment Model

Acceptance and commitment model[23,24] integrates covert conditioning, where imagination behaviour therapy methods are used—the latter being primarily mindfulness and cognitive behaviour therapy. This model emphasizes the cognitive misinterpretations of pain and considers psychological inflexibility or rigid thought processes to be the cause behind the inability to lead a fairly normal life and engage in long-term beneficial goals. The intention of Acceptance and Commitment Therapy (ACT) is not to remove the distressful feelings, but rather to accept what has been given to us in this lifetime and to move towards valued goals. ACT helps the person to face the unpleasant feelings instead of negating them; it insists that such situations should not be avoided and teaches not to overreact to unpleasantness. Once the person learns to confront rather than avoid painful situations, it leads to some kind of 'workability' towards living a meaningful and valued life.

The ACT model believes that suffering is caused when the person has direct experience of control of behaviour through the interaction between distorted thoughts and emotions. In other words, pain hurts but the struggle with pain is what causes suffering.

Thus, the ACT model suggests a reverse strategy to manage pain. Its basic premise is that pain may be unpleasant, but while trying to manage it, one's living of life cannot be deferred. Many a time, controlling the pain by the patient maybe harmful, both physically and emotionally, because a rigid mindset prevents alternative thinking and promotes pain ruminations. This viewpoint is diametrically opposite to other models' explanation of chronic pain. Most models have concentrated upon distorted thoughts, alleviation of distress and suffering by enhancing mood states. The ACT model, on the other hand, focuses on acceptance of pain and the commitment to carry on living a meaningful life. The premise of this model is that instead of wasting time and efforts in trying to find a cure for pain or ways of controlling it, the focus should be on living life pursuing one's valued and cherished goals.

To do so, psychological inflexibility needs to be reduced. The transition from psychological inflexibility to flexibility requires travelling a mental and emotional journey that involves certain adjustments in one's cognitions, emotions and behaviour. Hence, psychological flexibility persuades the sufferer to stop trying to control pain and learn to face the unpleasant experience of pain as a part of life. The patient is not encouraged to *change* the thoughts or emotions about the pain, but is rather helped to *confront* the unpleasant thoughts, emotions, experiences, memories and sensations from the standpoint of acceptance and as a reality of life. The basic idea is not to negate the unpleasantness but to face and accept it. Psychological flexibility allows the person to commit to a behaviour that has a valued end. This helps in minimizing and then preventing the ruminations of pain thoughts that had, hitherto, been intimidating and restricting meaningful activities.

Psychological flexibility is maintained by the six concepts of ACT: a) acceptance, b) cognitive defusion, c) being present, d) self as context, e) values and f) committed action. Let us examine each concept a little in detail.

The first step to the therapeutic strategy of ACT model is acceptance that there is a problem and that the problem is pain and that I can willingly bear it. Pain is not to be considered as an adversary that needs to be controlled, fought or even stopped. Instead of trying to constantly escape pain, the person needs to learn to accept it as a normal part of life and instead of struggling with it, try to engage in some meaningful activities. The goal of the therapy also encompasses the unpleasant feelings that pain generates. Even distress, one of the offshoots of pain, is not suppressed but acknowledged as part of the goal.

Cognitive defusion literally means separation of emotion provoking stimulus from the unwanted emotional response—in this case, the emotional pain response. The analogy of defusing a bomb or a crisis comes to mind as being similar to cognitive defusion. In order to defuse the thoughts, the aim should not be to challenge, change or control them but, rather to recognize it as any other ordinary thought. The idea is to only modify the undesirable thoughts rather than alter the frequency, form or situation sensitivity that instigates the pain response. Simply put, it means that an endeavour is made to change the way one interacts or relates to one's thought by forming a different context so that the dysfunctional behaviour and emotions attached to the thoughts get minimized. This gives the person the leverage to choose not to be affected or influenced by it. Through the defusion process, the person learns to reduce the believability of the painful thoughts and thereby differentiates between thoughts and what constitutes as truth or reality.

Being present involves non-judgemental relations with the past events and being involved, more crucially, with the current ongoing psychological events happening in the environment. Thus, the person is encouraged to remain in the present instead of replaying past events in their mind or worrying about possible future sufferings. Help is given to focus on the here and now moment, in real time, consciously paying attention to the present. The intention is to promote a direct interaction with the environment, so that the person experiences the world in the present moment. Language used by the patient should be only to describe and note the pain-related events, and not to sound judgemental and deterimental to oneself. This endorses flexibility in behaviour and helps maintain the cherished values.

Self as context is the visualization of self being the locus or an identity that is more important than the thoughts, emotions or even the physical body. This helps in viewing self by becoming self-aware and being conscious of the present moment. In other words, it reflects viewing self as if from outside or objectively, that is 'observer self' or 'self as context'. This objectivity changes the person's perspective and only then is one able to challenge what one has become. For instance, when pain and person become inseparable, the visualization of self as context helps the person to separate themselves from pain by observing their pain without becoming their own pain.

Values are the chosen activities that the person is encouraged to pursue. Fear of pain usually limits the person's valued pursuits like occupation, relationships or even simple activities like taking a walk, playing with children and participation in festivities. When the set values and their implementation get aligned, they add meaning to the life of the patient.

Committed Action, as the words denote, is the patient's commitment to modify their behaviour by doing actions that promote their values in spite of their pain. Let us illustrate this point with an example. A person who values learning may be encouraged to learn something new like a musical instrument or language, or a person who likes to mingle with people and make new friends is encouraged to socialize. Since these are meaningful and purposeful activities, it facilitates the person to focus more in living their lives than ruminating constantly about their pain.

ACT model assists the chronic pain patient to accept experiences rather than reject them for the fear of pain. The aid provided is to choose behaviour mindfully using mindfulness techniques after giving it full attention instead of struggling with their previous conditioned or automatic responses. These steps help in improving the quality of life of a chronic pain patient.

~

Mrs Vandy was diagnosed with rheumatoid arthritis when she was forty-two years old. Three years of illness with frequent exacerbations had affected her both physically and mentally. When she initially approached us for therapy, she had expressed fear of pain, of frequent exacerbations of the illness, fear of deformity and, above all, of disability. She confided that although she had a very supportive family, her fear of disability remained extremely high because she had always been an active and independent person. When asked what disability meant to her, she replied that it was dependence on others and lack of dignity. She was depressed that her illness would take away so many cherished activities that she had striven for all her life. When encouraged to reveal these dreams, she told us about her own ambitions for her talented daughters, her wish to write and travel. But she was worried that her illness would make her twisted and deformed, ugly and a burden. Since pain was constantly present, she doubted her capacity to continue working and was even apprehensive about the cost of the treatment. She also felt shattered since no other family member had a similar illness, nor did she know how she had gotten it. For countless hours, she had researched on the internet to find the reason for developing rheumatoid arthritis but had come up with no concrete answers. She confessed that for the first time her thoughts centred on whether God was being punitive and punishing her. Losing her faith in God was the last straw. She expressed her anguish in these words: 'A tsunami has wiped my life's slate clean and written one word on it—misery.'

The radiological reports showed that the illness was not advanced and the pathological reports also showed that the inflammatory markers were well under control, which was good news for her. The pain appeared to be more in her mind than in her body. The ACT model was the correct choice of therapy for her. Since she already had certain well-defined goals in her mind, they were used as values to be lived and striven for despite the pain. The therapy concentrated on the here and now moment, that is, learning to live in the present. Suggestions were made to keep her meaningfully occupied instead of constantly being vigilant about swelling on her hands or reacting to every twinge of pain in the body. She was also dissuaded from doing any further research on the cause for the illness. As therapy progressed, the emotional reaction to the disease, hypervigilance for signs of inflammation, constant thoughts of disability and fear of sustaining injury reduced. She was encouraged to pursue writing, and that had a cathartic effect on her. Follow-ups even after a decade of the therapy sessions revealed that she continues to write extensively (her cherished goal), was able to nurture her daughters (both accomplished their respective goals) and at the same time she also preserved her own well-being. Despite exacerbations, she is able to cope with the illness in a positive manner without getting unduly distressed. Hence, ACT—acceptance of the disease and commitment towards self, by improving her functionality and reducing her distress—had actually ameliorated the chronic condition and produced remarkable results.

As we have seen, chronic pain and psychological disorders can not only coexist, but there is also a bidirectional relation between the two. Many chronic pain patients and their families do not realize that physical injury or pain can have a huge psychological impact on the life of the patient, which, in turn, leads to the chronicity of pain. An injury that refuses to yield to treatment brings in its wake a plethora of mangled thoughts, emotions and behaviour, which themselves ultimately culminate to form another disease—chronic pain.

4

Risk Factors for Chronic Pain

The experience of pain in human beings shows a great deal of inter-individual variability. All kinds of pain do not become chronic and neither do all persons with minor or major injuries experience chronic pain. Some cannot tolerate even a tetanus toxoid injection, while others can go through the pain of childbirth with great fortitude. How can this difference be explained? Can we identify the risk factors that predispose one person to suffer pain and spare another?

This can mostly be explained as interplay of nature versus nurture. Our nature, which includes our genes and other biological factors, are inherent in us and cannot be changed, hence, are non-modifiable risk factors. On the other hand, nurture or environmental factors can be modified, either increased or decreased, hence are modifiable risk factors.

Non-modifiable risk factors include age, gender, genetic predisposition, ethnicity, comorbidities, history of trauma (physical or psychological), socio-economic and cultural background. Modifiable risk factors include lifestyle factors, mental health and psychological factors, employment status and other occupational factors and control of comorbidities. Pain is also a modifiable risk factor. Untreated pain arising from any source, such as surgery or injury, can itself predispose one to develop chronic pain.

However, the divide between modifiable and non-modifiable risk factors is not cast in iron and this makes the interplay between them rather complex. For example, diabetes, heart and lung diseases may be non-modifiable risk factors, but the effects that they have on the body, and on pain in particular, can be modified by taking appropriate treatment, making lifestyle changes and, in the case of diabetes, maintaining tight glycaemic control. Trauma (accidents or surgery) and stress (physical and psychological), though unavoidable, can be managed to a large extent with the help of adequate treatment and, hence, are also modifiable risk factors.

Let us now discuss some of the non-modifiable risk factors that predispose one to develop chronic pain.

Non-modifiable Risk Factors

Age

Though pain is experienced at all ages, chronic pain is most often associated with advanced years due to the degenerative changes that occur with ageing and the presence of increasing comorbidities. The relationship between chronic pain and old age is not linear, but its prevalence is seen most in those above 65 years of age. In a comparative study of three groups of people ranging from 18–39 years, 40–59 years and 60–81 years, chronic pain was reported higher (31.2 per cent) in the third group, as compared to the others.[1] The occurrence of certain types of neuropathic pain is greater in elderly people. For instance, the incidence of post-herpetic neuralgia, which is a painful condition that occurs after herpes zoster (shingles), is associated with increased pain in the elderly population as compared to younger people.

With the increase in life expectancy and the likelihood of many more persons reaching the eighth and ninth decade, it is to be expected that the incidences of chronic pain would be high. On the other hand, lifestyle factors and stress, both at the workplace and at home, could be causes of elevated incidences of pain in the younger population. In a recent study spanning forty-two countries, it was found that 20.6 per cent of adolescents reported chronic pain—mainly headaches, backaches and stomach aches.[2]

Gender

Women have been found to have a lower threshold of pain, less tolerance for pain and experience more incidences of pain and analgesic sensitivity as compared to men.[3,4] The prevalence of chronic pain conditions—such as fibromyalgia, migraine, temporomandibular joint dysfunction and irritable bowel syndrome for instance—has been found to be much higher in women. In the authors' personal experience, too, the previous year's pain OPD (outpatient department) statistics revealed that more women (71.6 per cent) presented with chronic pain compared to men (28.4 per cent).

This gender difference could have both biological and psychological basis. Biologically, men and women differ. The hormonal changes that women experience at the time of puberty and menopause, involving oestrogen levels may be partly contributory although this has not been fully substantiated. Psychologically, it has been observed that those women who have poor coping strategies experience more chronic pain.[5]

Mrs Chandra, aged 64 years, presented at the Pain Clinic with severe shooting pain on the right side of her face which radiated to the tongue, back of her mouth and the right ear making it difficult for her to swallow solid food. It was diagnosed as right glossopharyngeal neuralgia, which is pain along one of the nerves originating in the brain. This nerve supplies the tongue, tonsils and the ear. Mrs Chandra had a history of depression and was anxiety prone, for which she was already on medications.

A combination of anticonvulsants, antidepressants and analgesics was started, which brought her relief from pain within a period of two months. Meanwhile, her husband fell severely ill, first with urinary tract infection and later with Covid-19. He was hosptalized both the times. Though her own pain had subsided and her husband had recovered completely from both illnesses, she continued to remain anxious. Her anxieties centred on her own pain resurfacing once her medications would be stopped and nebulous worries about her husband's health. Since she was a worrier, anticipatory anxiety was high, indicating anxiety sensitivity and pain catastrophic tendencies.

Genetic Factors: Nature or Nurture

Pain sensitivity and tolerance to pain are to a large extent determined by our genes, and there is a definite link between heredity and a number of pain conditions. There is no known unique gene for pain, but a multifarious combination of genetic factors—interacting with psychological, social and lifestyle factors—act at multiple levels in the development, processing and perception of pain. The underlying mechanism is not yet well or fully understood.[6,7,8,9]

At present there are more than 150 genes associated with chronic pain and this number is increasing. This is especially true for migraine, back and neck pain and chronic widespread pain like fibromyalgia. The likelihood of heritability of migraine, chronic tension type headaches and fibromyalgia maybe as high as 50 per cent. That of low back pain is estimated to be 46 per cent. In a study on twins (as that could assess the influence of genetics), it was found that genetics contributed to 21–67 per cent of back pain.[10] In fact, birth cohort studies have shown that chronic pain conditions 'run in families' so that children of parents with chronic pain conditions are more likely to develop chronic pain.[11]

However, behaviourists have emphasized the role of learning being equally important when pain runs in families. Children who see parents in pain but see them exhibiting no desire to get better, using pain as an excuse to shirk responsibilities, learn from them that pain behaviour can be used as a coping strategy to deal with life's difficulties. Furthermore, those children, who have strong identification with the parent in pain, are likely to exhibit pain behaviour as an adult.

Socioeconomic Status

Two aspects of socioeconomic status (SES) are of significance as contributing to pain—*social,* which includes education, community standing and neighbourhood of residence; and *economic,* which is represented by financial and material wealth. SES has been particularly linked to musculoskeletal pain and headaches.

Chronic pain and SES are inversely related. This indicates that people with lower social and economic stability are likely to experience more chronic pain and with greater severity. It is possible that financial restrictions, lower education, income inequalities, neighbourhood deprivation, fewer employment opportunities and lesser resources all add up to make a person anxious and depressed leading to poor coping mechanisms. The reverse could also be equally true. When the SES is high, the person has plenty of resources for maintaining an income for a comfortable life and adequate treatment opportunities and consequently there are lesser chances of chronicity of pain and emotional distress.[12]

SES is important insofar as it provides better means to deal with chronic pain. It certainly does not make anyone immune to chronic pain, and chronic pain does not really spare anyone belonging to any background from its clutches.

Ethnicity and Cultural Background

Cultural beliefs, traditions and ethnicity also influence pain experiences. Although risk factors may be consistent across cultures for chronic pain, its expression, perception, coping behaviour and management may differ. Experimental studies using multiple pain stimuli on different ethnic groups showed that Asians, African Americans and Hispanics showed lower pain tolerance as compared to Whites.[13] This indicated that pain sensitivity differed in different ethnic groups making ethnicity a risk factor for developing chronic pain.

Prior Surgery

In some patients, pain at the site of a previous surgery can persist long after the healing process is over and may last for months and even years. This condition is called chronic post-surgical pain (CPSP) and happens when acute post-surgical pain transitions to chronic pain. Its incidence varies from as low as 5 per cent to as high as 85 per cent.[14] Factors that contribute to this condition include female gender, young age, genetic predisposition and pre-existing psychosocial issues. Some heritable comorbidities like fibromyalgia, irritable bowel syndrome, irritable bladder, backache and migraine can predispose to CPSP. An important cause for CPSP is unrelieved postoperative pain, as we saw in Rahul's case in the first chapter. The most common surgical causes for chronic pain are associated with orthopaedic, breast, chest, heart, knee replacement surgeries and hernia repair.

Interestingly, those individuals who had severe perioperative anxiety, an emotional disposition and negative thoughts associated with surgery and its outcome, felt more traumatized making them more susceptible for CPSP.

Physical and Psychological Trauma

A prior history of trauma is another risk factor for chronic pain. Post-traumatic stress disorder (PTSD), an anxiety disorder, is a set of reactions after a person has been through some traumatic experience. Amongst the many types of traumas, the experiences of violence (physical, verbal or sexual) are most strongly related to chronic pain. Since the memories are so painful, any cues or reminders of the event provided by people, place, activities, thoughts or feelings, can provoke physical and psychological pain. Patients with PTSD are likely to develop chronic pelvic pain (e.g., painful bladder syndrome), low back pain, facial pain, fibromyalgia and non-remitting whiplash syndromes.[15]

For several decades, sexual abuse and parent-child interaction have been linked to pain behaviour.[16] Children who have faced physical abuse or sexual abuse—particularly a girl child—would grow up with feelings of inadequacy, low self-esteem, anxiety and somatic complaints. Children who find their otherwise cold and distant parents become caring, attentive and showing warmth when they were in pain, soon learn that 'pain and suffering gains love'. These parents inadvertently endorse pain behaviour in their child. Such children grow up legitimizing pain by internalizing pain cues and behaviours and, on any sign of stress and distress, can experience pain. The prevalence of chronic pain in PTSD can vary from 1–23 per cent.

Having discussed the non-modifiable risk factors for chronic pain let us now look at some of the modifiable risk factors.

Modifiable Risk Factors

Pain

Perhaps pain itself is the biggest risk factor for chronic pain. This applies to both acute and chronic pain. The more severe the acute pain, the more the chances of it developing to chronicity.[17,18] This is especially seen in patients who sustain injury following accidents or experience unrelieved postoperative pain (CPSP).

Interestingly, a recent study in humans has shown that repeated painful stimuli bring changes in the structure of the brain—especially in the areas responsible for sensing pain. These changes are reversible if the painful stimuli are stopped, as seen in both acute and chronic pain.[19] This raises issues regarding remodelling of the brain or the structural plasticity of the brain (neuroplasticity). The fact that these changes are reversible further gives impetus to early and adequate management of pain following trauma or surgery. This not only alleviates pain and distress but can also prevent its transition into chronicity.

Mental Health

Mental health and chronic pain run parallel to each other. We already know that the pain circuit in the brain is in close proximity to the emotional circuit (limbic system) and, therefore, chronic pain does precipitate psychological disturbances. In fact, chronic pain and psychological disorders have a bidirectional relationship, one affecting the other. Amongst the constellation of symptoms in many psychological disorders, one of the symptoms could be pain. Thus, psychological reasons tend to compound an already distressing situation.

Let us discuss some of the psychological disorders that predispose to chronic pain.

Depression

Chronic pain and depression have a strong bidirectional relationship. Major depression is characterized by certain distorted thoughts that aggravate the pain condition. Catastrophizing, which is an exaggerated negative thought about the worst happening, creates either an anticipation of occurrence of an actual pain condition or worsening of an already existing one. Catastrophizing thoughts heighten the pain experience, which, in turn, exacerbates the negative mood states, adding on to an already stressful situation and poor physical functioning. In the specific painful conditions of fibromyalgia, chronic abdominal pain, chronic spinal pain and temporo-mandibular joint disorders, the prevalence of depression can be as high as 50 per cent.[20,21,22]

Low-level chronic depression or dysthymia is very often seen in chronic pain patients. The prevalence of dysthymia is 1–9 per cent.[23] It can be incapacitating as it can increase perception of stress, reduce ability to cope with day-to-day problems, increase interpersonal relationship conflicts, affect the quality of life and may even lead to substance abuse or dependence and suicidal thoughts.

Depression of any kind makes a person emotionally fragile and thoughts of ending one's life are a common occurrence. Suicidal behaviour includes varied experiences from 'life weariness' or passive suicidal ideation to active suicidal thoughts and intentions to completed suicide. Suicidal thoughts are strongly related to depression, severe or recurrent headaches, psychogenic pain and abdominal pain.

Anxiety

Anxiety disorders are a group of psychological conditions that include generalized anxiety disorder (GAD), panic attacks, phobias (including agoraphobia, in particular), obsessive-compulsive disorder and post-traumatic stress disorder (PTSD). Broadly speaking, anxiety is feeling of apprehension or fear that something 'bad' is going to happen. Certain anxiety disorders like GAD, panic attacks, agoraphobia and PTSD, in particular, can be risk factors for chronic pain. The first three disorders are briefly discussed below.

Generalized anxiety disorder (GAD)

This is a condition in which the person is constantly plagued with excessive worries about a number of different things. The worries can range across any issue, be it health, work, family, finances or even very small concerns that most people would normally overlook. In the previously cited case of Mrs Chandra, excessive worry about the health of both her husband and herself was seen.

Persons with GAD are anxiety-sensitive. Constant arousal is interpreted as catastrophic, making one hypervigilant for any threat. This lowers the alarm threshold that triggers further anxiety and thereby enhances the intensity of pain. Over a period of time, it becomes difficult for a person to distinguish between actual chronic physical pain and anxiety-related pain.[24] The prevalence of GAD in chronic pain ranges from 1–10 per cent.[25]

Panic attacks

These are sudden episodes of intense fear that trigger severe anxiety, even when there may be no apparent reason or imminent danger. In pain patients, panic attacks could, for instance, be related to the fear of pain itself, increased intensity of pain, fear of procedures that are painful and even physical exercises. Since distress is high, it prompts the person to avoid those situations that are perceived as being the reason for the panic attack. Panic attacks in chronic pain patients range from 1–28 per cent.[26]

Agoraphobia

This is the fear or avoidance of places or situations where one may feel trapped, helpless or embarrassed. Normally, agoraphobia and panic attacks are seen together because an association develops between a particular place or a situation and panic attacks. These situations may be places associated with pain for the patient. It can be the hospital, the doctor's clinic or the doctor too. It could also be the place of a prior accident or anything that reminds the person of pain or painful experiences. Fears associated with an inability to escape from the situation could actually intensify anxiety. Agoraphobia is seen in 1–8 per cent of patients with chronic pain.[25]

Other significant mental disorders influencing chronic pain

Bodily distress disorder

This is the new name given to Somatoform Disorders (Pain Disorder) in ICD-11 [*International Classification of Diseases*, 11th Revision] and Somatic Symptom Disorder in DSM-5 [*Diagnostic and Statistical Manual of Mental Disorders*, 5th Ed.]. It is characterized by the presence of bodily symptoms that are distressing to the individual. There may be a single symptom, usually pain or fatigue, or there maybe multiple symptoms. The individual pays excessive attention to these physical symptoms and repeatedly consults various healthcare providers.

Personality characteristics and disorders

Certain personality types and personality traits can be predisposing factors for chronic pain. These include the trait of neuroticism and several personality disorders. Persons with high neuroticism are more likely to be moody, anxious, easily angered and frustrated, have proneness toward developing guilt feelings, envy, jealousy, fear, worry and loneliness. Chronic pain patients with high neuroticism show a tendency towards higher reactivity to pain, greater pain-related anxiety, feeling intense pain-related suffering, being passive and unable to use problem-focused coping mechanisms. Consequently, they suffer from greater disability and poorer quality of life.

Personality disorder is a pervasive maladaptive way of thinking about oneself, others and the world.[27] As mentioned in the earlier chapter, certain personality disorders, particularly cluster B (Dramatic types) and cluster C (Avoidant Fearful types) are most closely associated with chronic pain. Both these clusters have high emotionality and poor self-perception.

Cluster B has four types of personality disorders: borderline, histrionic, narcissistic and antisocial personalities. Borderline personality disorder, which is characterized by high impulsivity, superficial and unstable relationships, emotional fluctuations and poor self-image, has a prevalence of chronic pain of 1–28 per cent. Histrionic personality disorder—associated with excessive emotionality, dramatic behaviours and attention-seeking behaviours—has a prevalence of chronic pain of 6–23 per cent. People with narcissistic personality disorder exhibit traits like grandiosity, self-love and high need for admiration and attention. The prevalence of chronic pain in these people ranges from 2–23 per cent. Persons with antisocial personality disorder have not shown a propensity towards chronic pain.

Amongst cluster C are grouped avoidant, dependent and obsessive-compulsive personality disorders. In this group two types, dependent and obsessive-compulsive, have shown strong correlation with pain behaviour. Dependent personality disorder is characterized by an excessive need to be cared for by others, poor confidence and decision-making abilities, submissiveness and fear of being alone. The prevalence of chronic pain in these people ranges between 2–17 per cent. Another disorder from this cluster, obsessive-compulsive personality disorder with hallmarks of perfectionism, orderliness, control and inflexibility has prevalence that ranges from 7–16 per cent.

Medical Comorbidities

Comorbidities present in a person can be both a non-modifiable or modifiable risk factor for chronic pain as mentioned in the beginning of the chapter. Generally speaking, the older the person, the more likely are the chances of comorbidities being present.

Let us first discuss some of the medical comorbidities that can predispose to chronic pain.

Neurological conditions

These include diseases related to the nervous system, either the brain, the spinal cord or the peripheral nerves. Patients with neurological illnesses like brain stroke, brain tumours, spinal-cord injury, multiple sclerosis (MS), trigeminal neuralgia and Parkinson's disease are prone to suffer from chronic pain. Nearly 8 per cent of people who suffer a brain stroke can have chronic pain and it is termed as central post-stroke pain. It could possibly be due to damage to the pain-conducting pathways in the brain as a result of stroke. Multiple sclerosis, a degenerative disease of the brain and spinal cord—which damages the insulating covers of the nerve cells (myelin sheath)—causes chronic pain in nearly 30 per cent patients. Parkinson's disease, which causes musculoskeletal problems like rigidity and stiffness and also dystonia (involuntary movements), can cause pain in nearly 40–80 per cent patients. In most of these neurological illnesses, pain is often associated with mood disorders (mainly depression), and both (the illness and the mood disorder) in conjunction can severely impact the quality of life.

Spinal-cord injury, a neurological condition due to a traumatic injury to the spine, causes pain in as many as 70 per cent patients, mostly in the younger age group. This pain (neuropathic pain) is usually burning or perhaps sharp and shooting in nature and may be associated with tingling, numbness and increased sensitivity of the skin. It can be excruciating, unrelenting and resistant to treatment modalities.

Patients with neurodegenerative/neurocognitive disorders like Alzheimer's disease can suffer from chronic pain, the incidences being as high as 45.8 per cent.[28] The main sources of pain in these patients are musculoskeletal (mainly knees and spine), the others being due to abdominal, gastro-intestinal, genito-urinary causes or due to wounds and pressure sores.

Certain diseases can affect the nerves in our body and can be a risk factor for chronic pain. One such medical condition is diabetes mellitus, an endocrine disorder in which high blood sugar levels damage nerves. It has been estimated that 50 per cent of patients with type 1 and type 2 diabetes are at risk for diabetic neuropathy. Since this is a very painful condition, it is referred to as painful diabetic neuropathy (PDN). In these patients, the distribution of pain, tingling and numbness is, characteristically, in the hands and feet in a 'glove and stocking' pattern.

Besides diabetes, long-term and heavy intake of alcohol, HIV infection and advanced kidney disease can also damage the peripheral nerves and cause painful peripheral neuropathy.

Comorbidities of the spine

As we are all aware, diseases of the spine, especially degenerative diseases, are an important cause of chronic pain. Fractures, cancers, inflammations and infections of the spine can also predispose to chronic pain.

Degenerative disease of the cervical spine, or cervical spondylosis, is one of the most common causes of neck and arm pain and may be associated with numbness in the arm, stiffness in the neck and even headaches. While in older patients pain emanating from the cervical spine is mainly due to degenerative changes, in younger people the cause may be due to infection, inflammation, injury or disc prolapse.

Mrs Yogita, a 48-year-old software engineer, had been having severe, incapacitating headaches for three years. She consulted a neurologist and, on her own insistence, asked for an MRI of her brain to be done. It revealed a small, benign brain tumour for which she underwent a brain surgery. Despite surgery there was still no relief in the intensity or frequency of the headaches. In fact, they only got worse. A repeat MRI of the brain ruled out any residual brain tumour or other abnormalities that could possibly contribute to the headaches.

When I examined her, I found that she had a rather rigid cervical spine with spasm in her neck and shoulder muscles. This was indeed a significant clinical finding. Blood tests that included HLA B27 and X-ray/ MRI of the cervical spine confirmed the diagnosis of spondyloarthropathy, which is an inflammatory condition of the ligaments and tendons of the spine. This had led to the rigidity of her cervical spine and could partially be the cause of her headaches, as some headaches, called cervicogenic headaches, originate from the tight muscles of the shoulders and cervical spine. The painful cervical spine had caused spasm of the muscles of her neck and led to headaches.

While in my Pain Clinic, I also observed an interesting facet in her behaviour. She appeared restless, was breathing hard and seemed unable to sit for long. This restlessness was suggestive of claustrophobia. Her agitation and distress warranted a detailed psychosocial evaluation.

Psychological testing indicated that she was an anxiety-prone person since her childhood. Her anxiety in closed places was so high that she preferred to stay in open spaces; so much so that even in winters, she would keep the doors of her room open with the fan on. Every day she would go for long drives for at least five to six hours to relieve her anxiety and headaches. In fact, while she was in the clinic, the door had to be kept open and even then she could not remain indoor for long. Headaches, difficulty in remaining indoors and hyperventilation became some of the reasons for social isolation.

Thus, besides spondyloarthropathy, this distraught lady was depressed, severely anxious and was suffering from claustrophobia—all of which were contributory factors for her increased pain.

Muscles and joint disease

Muscle disorders can be a major contributor to chronic pain and nearly 85 to 93 per cent of patients presenting to pain clinics have some kind of muscle involvement. Muscle spasm and rigidity can be the major underlying cause for chronic back pain, neck and shoulder pain, headaches, arm and leg pain and even abdominal and pelvic pain. Tight muscles can, in addition, entrap the nerves lying in their vicinity to cause neuropathies with burning or shooting pain, tingling, numbness and increased sensitivity to touch and pain. Myofascial pain syndrome (MPS) is a frequently encountered condition where muscles and its surrounding fascia (connective tissue) have taut bands or nodules in them, which can be very tender (myofascial trigger points).

Joint inflammation or arthritis is another important risk factor for chronic pain. The most common types of arthritis are degenerative arthritis (osteoarthritis) and inflammatory arthritis. The prevalence of osteoarthritis increases with age and nature of work and is more common in women. In a recent study its prevalence in the Indian population was found to be 28.7 per cent.[29] The non-modifiable risk factors for osteoarthritis include age, gender (more common in women), genetics, ethnicity and previous history of injury to the joint. The modifiable risk factors include obesity, type of occupation, sports injury and weakness of muscles around the joint due to lack of exercise.

The other type of arthritis, which contributes to pain and disability, is the inflammatory type, the prototype of which is rheumatoid arthritis. Here the body's immune system goes awry and mistakenly attacks the person's own joints causing inflammation. Hence, this is an autoimmune disease, which means that the body's natural defence mechanism cannot distinguish between its own cells and foreign cells. The prevalence rate in the general population is 1 per cent. It is more common in women, peaking between the ages of 35 to 50.

Whatever the cause for arthritis, its two cardinal features, pain and disability, can affect the personal, emotional and social life of the afflicted person.

Cancer

Cancer pain can be debilitating and distressing. In fact, the first fear that crosses the mind of the patient after diagnosis of cancer is not the fear of death but about the severity of pain they are likely to suffer. This is not a wholly unwarranted fear, as the incidences of pain in patients with cancer is between 30–50 per cent and in advanced stages it rises to 75–90 per cent. Besides the pain caused by cancer itself, treatment for cancer, especially chemotherapy, can be yet another cause of chronic pain. This is because the chemotherapy drug, besides destroying the cancer cells, also damages the nerves in the extremities. Hence, it is called chemotherapy-induced peripheral neuropathy (CIPN). Most often this pain is reversible after chemotherapy is stopped, but in some cases it can be irreversible and nearly 33 per cent of cancer survivors complain of this type of neuropathic pain.

Pelvic pain

An often underdiagnosed and overlooked cause of chronic abdominal pain that causes great distress and suffering is chronic pelvic pain.

The various conditions that can cause chronic pelvic pain are pelvic inflammatory disease, endometriosis, interstitial cystitis (painful bladder syndrome), irritable bowel disease and infections of the genitourinary tract. Chronic pelvic pain is more commonly seen in women, mainly because of the anatomic, physiological, hormonal and psychological differences between the two genders.

Employment Status and Occupation

Lack of employment or fears related to employability is a life event stressor for a person. Employment gives financial stability and, psychologically, a sense of security and the belief that one is a useful and productive member of the family and society. Unfortunately for chronic pain patients, loss of job or worry about loss of job creates fears and anxieties about being unemployed, having lower income, being relegated to a subordinate position and reduced prestige. This engenders negative thinking, particularly catastrophic thinking, that increases pain. Depression and low self-esteem are usually the fallout of fears related to employment.

Even the workplace scenario can impact pain. Most chronic pain patients are sceptical about sharing problems related to their pain with their employers, as it is a double bind situation. Being open about their condition belittles their creditability and decreases the chances of promotions and retention of the job. An unsympathetic employer often has the belief that conditions like fibromyalgia or chronic fatigue syndrome are nothing but laziness and sham or pretentious behaviour, as there are no obvious reasons for pain. Sympathy and consideration are often reserved for only those patients who have the so-called 'justifiable pain', as after surgery or accidents.

On the other hand, an employer's positive attitude helps in negotiating the amount of workload, hours of work, allocating flexible timings and providing adjustment in case of absenteeism. The employer's repose of faith and sympathy could be rewarded by the employee's renewed efforts to recover, maintain an optimistic stance and even more productivity.

Let me cite the example of a young medical resident doctor, Aarushi, working in a leading hospital. She had fibromyalgia along with dysthymia (chronic depression) and severe anxiety. During the Covid-19 pandemic, the hospital was busier than usual and she had to endure long working hours and frequent night duties. She tried her utmost to cope with the heavy work despite her pain. In spite of being aware of her chronic pain, her immediate boss, who was in charge of the duty roster, was rather inconsiderate while assigning duties. He often made insensitive remarks about her pain and on one such occasion even told her she was not fit for the job and that she should consider taking up some lighter work elsewhere. He even had the temerity to tell her that the pain was all in her head. Such inconsiderate behaviour and insensitive remarks would further upset and stress her, leading to frequent pain exacerbations. The head of the department, however, knowing her sincerity and conscientiousness, was not only compassionate but often intervened to allot her lighter duties.

Lifestyle Factors

In recent years attention has been paid to the role played by lifestyle factors in the genesis and maintenance of pain. Their importance was felt more seriously during the Covid-19 pandemic, which led to drastic changes in our lifestyle, some good and some not so good. These changes, in turn, have had repercussions on our body as well as on our mind.

Let us discuss some of these factors.

Physical activity and exercise

We are aware that a sedentary lifestyle is a risk factor for non-communicable diseases like diabetes, hypertension, stroke and some cancers. It could also be a risk factor for chronic pain conditions, especially musculoskeletal disorders like back pain, migraine, fibromyalgia and chronic fatigue syndrome. It has been seen that pain increases when physical activity is avoided and decreases with increase in activity levels, making it a bidirectional relationship. A sedentary lifestyle with lack of physical activity and exercise is often due to sheer laziness, lethargy or lack of motivation. In a majority of older adults, slowing of physical activity is a natural phenomenon. But many times, especially in patients with pain, it could be due to 'kinesiophobia', which is fear of movement. This could be either due to a genuine fear or it may just be a pain-avoidance behaviour.

The Covid-19 pandemic lockdown led to inadvertent curtailing of both physical activity and exercises, and that resulted in many more incidences of musculoskeletal pain in all age groups.

Obesity

An abnormal collection of fat in the body is called overweight and excessive fat is called obesity. A body mass index (BMI) of more than 25 is considered overweight and above 30 is obesity. Obesity becomes a risk factor for chronic pain. Many chronic pain conditions like low back pain, osteoarthritis, headaches, chronic widespread pain like fibromyalgia, abdominal and pelvic pain, neuropathic pains and even musculoskeletal conditions like tennis elbow have been associated with obesity.

Obesity increases the mechanical load on the body by causing a higher compressive force and increased shear on various weight-bearing structures such as the lumbar spine and joints like the hip and knees. This, in turn, accelerates the degenerative changes and predisposes to pain and disability. Also, in obese people, adipose tissue, which is the loose connective tissue that stores fat, is believed to have a high concentration of inflammatory mediators such as cytokines and chemokines. These are important chemical mediators in the transmission of pain and, thus, possibly contribute to a pro-inflammatory state. Moreover, obese people are more likely to be kinesiophobic. All these factors can predispose them to various types of chronic pain conditions.

Posture

Bad posture is another risk factor for back pain, headache, neck and shoulder pain besides having an adverse effect on the balance of our body, on our mood, cardiovascular health and respiratory function. Bad posture is a faulty relationship of the body parts making it susceptible to strain and less efficient balance of the body over its support base.

An increasing number of youngsters are presenting with chronic neck and shoulder pain. The postural factors contributing to this include prolonged bending of the neck and sitting hunched over computers and laptops, prolonged use of cellphones, heavy backpacks and, in general, poor ergonomics. Poor posture could contribute to low back pain and nearly 25–51 per cent of office-goers, who sit for long durations, experience low back pain.[30] Sitting for long durations at a time can decrease the normal lumbar curvature, increase pressure on the intervertebral disc and can predispose to disc prolapse.

Sleep

Sleep deprivation impacts health by causing fatigue, mood changes, cognitive disturbances, anxiety and depression, all of which can worsen pain. Disrupted sleep could be a risk factor for chronic pain by lowering the pain threshold and pain tolerance. On the other hand, pain can lead to sleep disturbance, which is directly linked to the intensity of pain. For every point rise on the 10-point visual analogue pain scale, the likelihood of sleep disturbance increases by 10 per cent. Nearly half the number of back pain patients (47 per cent) have been found to report insomnia.[31] Similarly, a large number of patients with chronic widespread pain, as in fibromyalgia, report disturbed and unrefreshed sleep. It is still not clear whether insomnia causes pain or vice versa, or is the link bidirectional. As mentioned earlier in chapter two, in the neuromatrix of pain in the brain, the neuroanatomy of pain and sleep pathways overlap and that could explain the link between pain and sleep.

Stress

Stress disturbs the equilibrium of both the mind and the body. Both life events or acute stress and daily hassles or chronic stress, have a bearing on pain behaviour. Of the two, chronic stress tends to be more debilitating. Chronic stress keeps the nervous system in a constant state of overdrive. This continuous activation increases the intensity of pain, which in itself becomes the reason for stress. Stress keeps the muscles tensed or in spasm, which further amplifies pain. This bidirectional relationship between stress and chronic pain was clearly evident during the Covid-19 pandemic.

Substance-use disorders

Alcohol use, its abuse and sometimes dependence is seen in persons with chronic pain. From ancient times, alcohol and its corrupted versions have been used as an analgesic or pain reliever. Though the effect of alcohol in relieving pain is only temporary, yet it is often utilized as self-medication by the sufferer. As tolerance to alcohol is easily developed, it needs to be taken in greater quantities to reduce the same degree of pain over time. It must also be kept in mind that severe pain is one of the withdrawal symptoms of chronic alcohol drinkers, which itself becomes a reason to continue drinking alcohol.

Smoking is seen more among chronic pain patients than the general population. Smokers can have pain in multiple areas of the body and also increased pain intensity as compared to non-smoking pain patients. There is a link between tobacco use and decrease in bone density (osteoporosis), which can also predispose to pain. It has been found that smoking not only affects the person physically by increasing pain intensity and causing fatigue and sleep disturbances, but is associated with adverse psychological effects such as pain behaviours, anger, need for emotional support, anxiety and depression. These repercussions manifest in *pain interference*, which implies that they interfere with the functioning at home, work or in the social environment. On the other hand, quitting smoking improves musculoskeletal health and exercise endurance by improving perfusion of blood to muscle and bones and preserving bone density.

Alcohol and other non-opioid abuse are highest among the sufferers of fibromyalgia, chronic spinal pain and arthritis; lowest among patients with migraine headaches and neuropathic pain. Overall, substance use ranges from 27–87 per cent in chronic pain patients.

Other Modifiable Risk Factors

Osteoporosis

Osteoporosis is a condition characterized by poor quality of bone and low bone density, which leads to increased bone fragility and risk for fractures. Although the pain seen with fractures is acute to start with, it can, over a period of time, become chronic leading to disability. Even without fractures, osteoporosis can, per se, cause pain in muscle and bones. There is an independent positive association between osteoporosis and back pain. Interestingly, males are more prone to osteoporosis-induced back pain.

How does osteoporosis impact the musculoskeletal system and predispose to pain? It does so by causing low bone mass and micro-architectural deterioration in bone tissues leading to bone fragility and even fractures. Insufficient central axial skeletal support, in turn, leads to imbalance of muscle and ligaments of the spine, which could bring structural changes in the curvature of the spine, disturb its biomechanics and even cause its instability. All these consequences of osteoporosis make the person vulnerable to chronic pain.

Vitamin deficiency

Vitamin D deficiency is among the most common nutritional deficiencies and is prevalent all over the world, including in sunshine-sufficient countries like India. Its high incidence in India (40–99 per cent) could probably be because of poor dietary intake, changing lifestyle, increased skin pigmentation and application of sunscreen as well as some cultural practices that require covering the entire body, such as wearing the burqa.[32]

Besides causing a whole range of conditions—ranging from skeletal problems to heart disease and cancer—it has been closely linked to the causation and maintenance of chronic pain. Inadequate levels of vitamin D can cause—by a combination of anatomical, hormonal, neurological and immunological effects—muscle, bone and joint pain, fatigue and muscle weakness. It has been found that people with chronic widespread pain, as well as 'other pain', were more likely to have vitamin D deficiency as compared to people who had no pain.[33]

The Impact of Covid-19 Pandemic on Pain

The Covid-19 pandemic witnessed a sea change in the lifestyle and mental health of people all over the world. The harsh lockdown, the fear of contracting the dreaded disease and the socioeconomic repercussions of the lockdown had a huge impact on the lives of people. Offices and workplaces were abandoned and work from home became the order of the day. While some people managed to create workstations nearly akin to what they were habituated to in office, a large majority could not or did not do so. They worked while sitting on beds, sofas or couches and placing laptops on their laps or bending forward to work on laptops placed on tables that were not of an appropriate height. Poor ergonomics like faulty posture, sitting without proper support for their back, neck or arms etc., took its toll and led to aches and pains that were predominantly musculoskeletal.

Physical burdens—that one was not used to before the pandemic—could also have predisposed people to pain. The increase in household chores due to the unavailability of domestic help, keeping the children occupied with studies as well as other extra-curricular activities and their own work-from-home duties only added to their woes. Combined with that sudden onslaught of work, was the lack of regular exercise, walks and working out in a gymnasium. Further augmenting the already existing troubles, were the rigours of disinfecting anything and everything coming from outside for fear of contracting the dreaded virus.

Mental health, too, took a major hit and an increase in anxiety and depression was witnessed during the pandemic like never before. The fear of getting infected, deaths in the family due to Covid-19 infection, loss of jobs, financial constraints, lack of social life and loneliness created tremendous stress. One important fear was related to the paucity of hospital beds for loved ones, shortage of essential medicines and non-availability of something as vital as oxygen if the need arose. Besides, many persons with chronic diseases like diabetes, cancer, arthritis and other pain conditions were unable to seek treatment and suffered in silence as they feared venturing out of the confines of their homes.

Prevailing conditions, no doubt, played havoc with the physical and mental conditions of nearly everyone in the world, but far more so among patients with any chronic disease. In chronic pain patients especially, the aftermath of lockdown had been severe. Many unprecedented changes like lack of exercise resulted in physical deconditioning, weight gain, no proper routine, worries of employability or re-employability and unexpected financial constraints. This had indeed given rise to mental distress in the form of increased fears, anxieties, depression and suicidal thoughts. These physical, mental and emotional health problems could have been responsible for the amplication of pain conditions witnessed in the last few years.

Let us now see how chronic pain impacts nearly every aspect of a person's life.

5

Physical and Psychological Impact of Chronic Pain

We have understood that chronic pain is debilitating and brings about undesirable changes to our body and mind. A plethora of devastating side effects are generated by chronic pain. These side effects become a source of discomfort and, in turn, affect many functions that are necessary for our day-to-day life to varying degrees. These changes create a circular, sometimes bidirectional, relationship, which compounds an already complex phenomenon of chronic pain.

Impact of Chronic Pain

The impact of short-lived pain, as seen in acute pain, is usually transient and ceases with cessation of pain. Chronic pain, on the other hand, can be all-pervasive and has an adverse impact on the functioning of the various systems of the body. Besides its effect on the nervous system and the locomotor system, it can affect other systems of the body such as the cardiovascular system, gastrointestinal system, the endocrine system, the immune system and, last but not the least, the mental health of the person. Since it involves all the aspects—physical, emotional and cognitive—pain management needs to be holistic, encompassing all aspects to be effective.

Let us look at a case study to understand the impact of chronic pain on the body and mind.

Mrs Indu was a 75-year-old woman weighing 90 kg, who had suffered from chronic back pain and sciatica for fifteen years. Since the past two years she had also complained of pain in both knees and had difficulty in balancing herself especially while walking. She had been to a spine specialist ten years ago and he had diagnosed her as having degenerative spine disease at multiple levels in the lumbar spine and had advised surgery. But she was unwilling to undergo surgery and had continued with conservative treatment such as medications and physiotherapy. Over the years she had even tried alternative medicines like homeopathy and Ayurveda, which only provided temporary relief. Pain in her lower back and legs continued, worsening over the years. Her unsteady gait even led to several falls. To prevent this, she initially used a walking stick for support, then a walker and since the last few months she had started using a wheelchair. Her increasing immobility led to weight gain and obesity. Besides, she felt extreme weakness and fatigue even doing mundane tasks. Her sleep, too, was disturbed because of pain.

She had also suffered from hypertension and diabetes for several years. Of late, despite taking insulin injections for her diabetes, her blood sugar levels had remained persistently high. Her blood pressure, too, was not well-controlled. She tended to get gastric acidity along with abdominal distension and also suffered from constipation.

Psychosocial history revealed significant findings. She had always been an anxious person to the point of being a worrier. She appeared depressed and repeatedly expressed her helplessness on being dependant on others for even simple needs. Her immediate caregivers were her son and daughter-in-law who were doing their utmost to take care of her. But being professionals themselves, they were not able to spend too much time talking to her or simply being with her. Her grandchildren, who were teenagers, had a busy schedule, oscillating between their studies and friends. Despite the presence of so many family members in her home, she felt lonely and neglected. Consequently, she became withdrawn and depressed, which further reduced her socializing activities with relatives and friends. Even activities like chopping vegetables, knitting and watching television serials, which she enjoyed doing earlier, had become a drudgery leaving her with no sense of enjoyment. Gradually she stopped participating in all these activities and started confining herself to her room and lying on her bed facing the wall. Often, she said, she cried herself to sleep and frequently thought of the futility of staying alive with so much of pain, loneliness, being a burden and a liability on her children.

She was on various medicines for her sciatica, which included anticonvulsants, antidepressants and analgesics. Besides her antihypertensive and diabetic medications, she was on sedatives to help her sleep along with drugs to counter gastric acidity and constipation.

Let us first discuss how chronic pain impacted Mrs Indu's physical health.

Locomotor System

The first and foremost impact of chronic pain on the body is on the locomotor system, which includes the skeleton, muscles, joints, tendons, ligaments and cartilage. Muscles can be a major contributor to chronic pain. Pain, whether acute or chronic, can cause splinting of muscles, which go into a spasm. This is, initially, a protective phenomenon to prevent further damage to the underlying structures, be it a fractured bone or an inflamed internal organ. But when the pain is long-lasting and chronic, the muscles can remain in a persistent state of contraction resulting in shortening of muscles as they do not go back to their original state of relaxation. Muscle shortening can result in pain and tenderness, especially when taut bands or knots (myofascial trigger points) are formed in the muscle. This condition is called myofascial pain syndrome. The tight muscles can limit movement and can result in painful joints as seen in arthritis. The resulting restriction in movement and even, at times, immobility, can lead to a chain of events. It can cause disuse atrophy of the muscles, which leads to a reduction in muscle bulk and wasting of the muscle thereby contributing to weakness, easy fatigability and further immobility. Furthermore, nerves can get trapped in the layers of contracted muscles leading to entrapment neuropathies, which can cause burning pain along with numbness and tingling sensations.

Immobility and inactivity, besides causing weakness and atrophy, can result in contractures and inflexibility of the body due to stiffness of muscles, tendons, ligaments and joints. It can lead to obesity which, in turn, can place a huge stress on joints and muscles by overloading them. The resulting wear and tear of the cartilage in the joints can further aggravate osteoarthritis of weight-bearing joints like the hip joint and knee joint. This endless cascade of events—wherein chronic pain causes inactivity, which then leads to muscle atrophy, obesity and further inactivity—is called 'physical deconditioning'.

In the case of Mrs Indu, the original problem started in the spine. Degeneration of the spine had led, over the years, to physical deconditioning, immobility and pain in other regions of the body as well. Thus, we see that pain begets pain.

Nervous System

When pain is persistent and long-lasting, sensory nerves from the affected area are constantly transmitting pain signals from the periphery towards the spinal cord and the brain. This constant onslaught of painful stimuli can cause a remodelling of the brain and the spinal cord, resulting in an augmentation in the central processing of the pain sensation. This phenomenon is called central sensitization, and the remodelling of the brain that occurs as a result is called neuroplasticity. Central sensitization and neuroplasticity cause the brain to become hypersensitive to even stimuli that do not normally cause pain, such as touch or a gust of wind. This has been discussed in detail in chapter 2.

Mrs Indu had age-related degeneration of the spine, which resulted in impingment of the nerves to the legs causing sciatica. In patients with sciatica, the pain originates from the lumbar spine (lower back) and radiates through the buttock and down the leg. It is usually due to compression of the sciatic nerve, which is the major nerve to the lower limbs. The common cause of sciatica is 'slipped' or herniated disc, but it can also happen due to age-related degeneration of the spine as we saw with Mrs Indu.

Fatigue and Stiffness

Fatigue and general weakness are common complaints in some patients with chronic pain conditions such as fibromyalgia, irritable bowel syndrome, rheumatoid arthritis, chronic tension headaches and even long-standing degenerative disease of the spine. Persistent fatigue is also the predominant symptom in a debilitating condition called chronic fatigue syndrome, also called myalgic encephalitis.

Fatigue in patients with chronic pain can be so troublesome that it considerably impairs even the day-to-day self-care activities; it is reported more often by women than men. Fatigue may partly be due to the other symptoms commonly associated with chronic pain such as insomnia, physical inactivity, obesity and poor diet. In fact, as mentioned earlier, lack of physical activity due to pain or pain-avoidance, can lead to disuse and atrophy of muscles which can cause physical deconditioning and fatigue as was seen in Mrs Indu.

Cardiovascular System

One of the systems adversely impacted by the stress response to pain is the cardiovascular system. This can predispose to hypertension, diabetes, dyslipidemia and obesity—all of which are risk factors for coronary artery disease and cardiac events. Also, increased anxiety in patients with chronic pain can cause palpitations and hypertension, which can lead to adverse cardiac events especially in the elderly and those with underlying heart disease.

Endocrine System

We know that any kind of stress impacts the endocrine system by eliciting a stress response with a rise in serum cortisol levels. However, excess cortisol secretion due to prolonged activation of the body's stress axis (hypothalamic-pituitary-adrenal axis), as in chronic pain, can adversely impact the endocrine system of our body and lead to hormonal imbalance and dysfunction. In such situations, there is a sustained rise in cortisol levels in the body, which can be harmful. One of the effects of high cortisol levels is glucose intolerance (high blood sugar) and increasing proneness to diabetes mellitus. Stress-induced high cortisol levels can also cause osteoporosis and, as mentioned earlier, hypertension, dyslipidemia and obesity.

When pain continues unabated, the body's stress axis can get over-stimulated resulting in the suppression of its normal function with the result that cortisol levels start declining to less than normal levels. Patients with low cortisol levels exhibit signs of dullness, apathy, weakness, weight loss, low appetite, muscle wasting, low blood pressure and insomnia. This is especially seen in chronic pain conditions like fibromyalgia, rheumatoid arthritis, chronic headaches, osteoarthritis and chronic fatigue syndrome.

Gastrointestinal System

Certain chronic pain conditions are often linked to gastrointestinal system disorders, especially irritable bowel syndrome (IBS, for this discussion). IBS is a functional gastrointestinal disorder which implies that there is no specific underlying cause for its occurrence. It is characterized by abdominal cramps, bloating and altered bowel habits such as diarrhoea or constipation, or both, and is a stress-sensitive condition. Pain, being a stressor, can often cause gastrointestinal upsets manifesting as IBS. Treating pain, by reducing stress and the stress response along with appropriate medications, can quite often control the symptoms of IBS.

The two most common chronic pain conditions associated with IBS are fibromyalgia and chronic pelvic pain (CPP). In fact, there are a lot of similarities between IBS and these two pain conditions. IBS is also found to be present in 70 per cent of patients with fibromyalgia. There is an overlap of symptoms in both conditions such as heightened pain sensitivity, sleep disturbances, mood disorders and easy fatigability. The other commonalities between these two conditions are that they are stress-induced and more frequently seen in women. The treatment for both are analgesics, antidepressants, anti-anxiety drugs along with behavioural therapy and psychotherapy.

Irritable bowel syndrome is encountered in one-third of all patients with CPP. In fact, many symptoms, both physical and psychological, are similar in IBS and CPP. The most common cause of CPP in women causing IBS is a gynaecological disorder, endometriosis.

Immune System

One of the systems that respond to a challenging situation to the body or a stressor is the immune system. Pain is one such stressor that activates our immune system. While both acute and chronic pain can affect the immune system, the effect of chronic pain on the immune system is more marked. This is because chronic pain causes long-term stress. With a consistent elevation of cortisol as well as pro-inflammatory cytokines, the immune system becomes resistant, exhausted and compromised. This could result in an increased susceptibility to infections and slow healing of wounds.

Indeed, researchers at the McGill University have found that genes in T cells are altered in chronic pain.[1] T cells are lymphocytes (a type of white blood cell) that are part of our body's adaptive immunity system and, hence, essential for our immunity. So, while acute pain activates our immune system and helps our immunity, chronic pain can depress it and make the person susceptible to illness and infection.

Looking back at Mrs Indu, let us see how chronic low back pain affected her physically.

The pain that originally started from the spine, gradually led to pain in other parts of the body because of the sequence of events that took place due to physical deconditioning. It was not just the pain of sciatica that was the cause of her distress, but the resulting muscle spasm, muscle atrophy, muscle weakness and obesity which had caused joint pains, instability and immobility resulting in a great deal of disability as well. This physical deconditioning contributed to her feeling of fatigue. Her biological functions, such as sleep and bowel habits, had also got disrupted. Besides, the overstress caused by long-standing pain had led to inadequate control of her blood pressure and blood sugar levels.

Psychological Impact

Let us now see how chronic pain impacts patients psychologically. This encompasses cognitive functions, emotions and interpersonal relationships. Each psychological component has a bearing on the other, which eventually has a cascading effect on the well-being of the person.

Impact of pain on cognitive functions

Attention, concentration and memory: Some cognitive functions that get impacted in chronic pain are attention, concentration and memory functions. 'Brain fog'—an inability to have a sharp focus and a good memory—is commonly reported in patients with fibromyalgia, which involves severe and widespread pain. Chronic depression and pervasive anxiety, which go hand-in-hand with chronic pain, are other reasons for cognitive disturbance. On the other hand, younger persons with chronic pain and those with less intensity of pain, report lower cognitive disturbances. There is greater likelihood of restoration of cognitive functions in these patients, as and when depression and pain intensity decrease, as we will see in the case discussed below.

Priya, a 28-year-old doctor, with a decade-old history of fibromyalgia with severe widespread body pains, extreme fatigue, disturbed sleep and depression, had simultaneously been experiencing poor concentration and short attention spans. She was preparing for her post-graduation entrance examination in medicine and found that she was unable to retain what she had studied and that eroded and undermined her self-confidence.

She described the experience as 'being in a haze'. She was started on a multi-pronged and multi-disciplinary therapy comprising medications, dry needling, graded physiotherapy as well as cognitive behaviour therapy for depression, following which her pain reduced substantially. Soon she was able to resume her hospital duties. When she also resumed her preparation for the entrance examination, not only was she able to concentrate better, but she also qualified in the examination.

Besides her physical and psychological symptoms, she had rightly spoken of experiencing 'brain fog' that hampered her studies. Amelioration of her pain and other symptoms improved her cognitive functions as well.

Attitude and beliefs: Attitudes and beliefs play a significant role in chronic pain. Beliefs are related to self-efficacy, i.e., belief in one's capability to succeed in a particular situation. When self-efficacy is high in chronic pain patients, there is perception of control in managing the pain experience, belief that the extent of harm and disability is manageable and not threatening and expectation of recovery is present. When self-efficacy is lacking, it makes a person feel helpless and vulnerable to either physical or psychological threats and is consequently related to poorer outcomes. Hence, the pre-existing attitudes and beliefs of patients with chronic pain have a profound impact not only on the prognosis and outcome, but even on the adherence and compliance to the treatment being administered.

Hopelessness, helplessness and powerlessness: Thoughts of hopelessness and helplessness are part of the depressive syndrome and dysthymia (chronic depression) and these are often seen in chronic pain patients. Hopelessness, as the very word connotes, is the feeling of despair that one's condition is unlikely to improve and is beyond hope. This may result in apathy, pessimism and learned helplessness. Learned helplessness occurs when someone enduring an adverse situation beyond her/his control, does *not* make an attempt to escape from it even when there is a clear and unambiguous chance to do so.[2] When a chronic pain patient develops learned helplessness, self-efficacy remarkably diminishes.

Mr Sharad, an 89-year-old retired Air Force officer had hitherto led a very active retired life. Besides going for long walks in a wooded area near his house, he also indulged in his favourite hobby of carpentry. He had converted the basement of his house into a workshop and would spend long hours making all kinds of furniture. But since the last couple of years, he had developed severe back pain with burning sensation in his legs. This had incapacitated him so much that he had to quit his walks and couldn't even go to the basement of his house. He was diagnosed with degenerative lumbar spine with neuropathic pain.

He had tried all types of allopathic treatment and alternative medicines like homeopathy and magneto therapy, but there had been no respite. An actively engaged octogenarian was now, unfortunately, confined to his house and much more to his bed, making him despondent, hopeless and helpless. Naturally, he became depressed and even had suicidal ideation. In fact, on his first visit to my Pain Clinic with his daughter, after narrating his history, he told me in despairing tones, 'I feel like jumping off my balcony and ending my life. I don't wish to live a vegetative life like this with so much pain.'

This elderly gentleman was depressed with feelings of hopelessness, helplessness and even suicidal ideation.

Powerlessness: This is another debilitating thought process and evokes the feeling that others have taken control of one's life and one has no control over one's body. In chronic pain patients, powerlessness is associated with thoughts of lack of control over the pain and the ensuing consequences on the body, and an inability to revert to their previously healthy states. Hopelessness, helplessness and powerlessness are predictors of poor outcomes for pain alleviation as the case below illustrates.

Geeta, a middle-aged woman, had fallen from her bed about eight months ago. She fell on her right side and although there were no fractures, she had sustained soft tissue injury on her right shoulder and hip. She also had bruises on her body, which were causing her discomfort and pain. Analgesics and physiotherapy failed to provide her relief. For most part of the last four months, she had complained of pain and refused to get off the bed. Initially, she was being carried around the house either by her son or a manservant, but eventually the family bought a wheelchair as she refused to walk.

Clinical examination and X-rays failed to reveal the reason for her inability to stand and walk. Since she had not been physically active, she had gained weight, which, in turn, was further aggravating the matter. She was referred for psychological evaluation, as the pain specialist found her looking depressed.

Her first statement to me, spoken rather defensively, was that she was mentally well although she felt sad about being confined to her bed. She firmly believed that her condition would never improve as nothing had helped her so far and that her case was hopeless. She described her family as irritating, as they kept pestering her to walk and move around when she could not even stand.

She was of the opinion that the doctors had missed the right diagnosis and she was powerless to do anything about it. Her moving words rather summed up her thoughts, 'I feel so powerless and helpless as no one is convinced of my pain, neither the doctors nor my family and, unfortunately, I have to depend on them.'

These negative thoughts were not allowing her to adhere to the treatment regimen and it was sabotaging her pain management.

Adjustment: Adjusting to changed circumstances and perhaps living with disability and constant pain is very challenging. By *adjustment* we mean the psychological processes through which people manage or cope with the demands and challenges of everyday life. A person suffering from chronic pain may be unable to fit with the environment, balance conflicting needs, operate effectively within their social setting and are likely to be riddled with stress and anxiety. In most cases, their *emotional adjustment* is poor and they may have difficulty in maintaining emotional equilibrium in the face of internal and external stressors. Let us now review in some detail how pain impacts emotions.

Emotional impact of pain

Guilt and shameful feelings: Each of us have a sense of right and wrong that is socially determined. When we believe, correctly or not, that we have compromised our standards of demeanour or morals in some way and feel responsible for the lacuna in demonstrating socially acceptable behaviour, we feel guilty. Guilt is akin to both remorse and shame. Remorse indicates guilt, regret and sorrow; shame is indicative of a negative evaluation of oneself.

Chronic pain and guilt have a strong correlation. Three types of pain-related guilt have been identified.[3,4] *Social guilt* is related to the inability to participate in social activities due to pain and, as a consequence, depriving family and friends of social occasions. This induces avoidance behaviour. *Pain guilt* is associated with either the inability to manage pain better or not putting enough effort to reduce pain. Lastly, *verification of pain guilt* is when in the absence of an actual cause, the patient tries to authenticate the pain by finding genuine reasons for the yet undiagnosed condition.

Shame is another negative feeling experienced by many a patient with chronic pain and disability. They may feel ashamed to be tended to, sometimes like babies. It can be demeaning for some patients when they have to seek assistance for wearing clothes, being fed and even for their daily ablutions. Some people with chronic pain feel ashamed of being a burden on family members and preventing them from living their own respective lives, as we saw in Mrs Indu's and Mrs Soma's cases.

Anger and blame towards self and others: Most persons with chronic pain feel frustrated and angry. This anger and frustration could be directed towards themselves, to their caregivers, towards the medical fraternity and sometimes to their own fate or even the Almighty. In fact, Dame Cicely Saunders,[5,6] in her concept of 'Total Pain', mentions spiritual pain, which means a person with cancer pain has negative existential thoughts and often questions and blames God or themselves for their suffering.

Thus, the reasons for anger in people with long-standing pain may be many, but it leaves in its wake a person who is dissatisfied, agitated and discouraged. It has been estimated that as many as 70 per cent of patients with chronic pain report feeling exceedingly angry most of the time.[7] Anger in chronic pain patients can range from irritation to blind rage. Their uncontrolled anger not only affects them psychologically but can also impact them physically, by increasing the intensity of pain and decreasing tolerance to pain. An emotionally upset and angry person invariably has poor sleep and higher chances of substance abuse (alcohol, cigarettes and drugs) and sometimes even comfort eating.

One middle-aged woman who had fibromyalgia said that if she did not eat to her satisfaction as soon as she felt hunger pangs, she would start crying. As a result, her children would immediately give her whatever food she liked in order to prevent her from getting upset. Even though she was a diabetic, she could not control her hunger and would eat foods rich in carbohydrates. This kind of comfort eating had further worsened her diabetic state, which further aggravated her pains.

An angry person would be more likely to experience interpersonal conflicts, social isolation and, in the long run, broken relationships.

Fears: Pain and fear go hand-in-hand, especially so in chronic pain. Several kinds of fears beset these patients, namely fear of increased pain, fear of disability and dependency and, in some, even fear of death. Fears of disability and death can get reinforced because of the gradual decline in physical, occupational, social and recreational activities of the person. Fear of death is especially seen in patients with cancer pain.

Fear in patients develops when even a beneficial activity like exercise causes the brain to interpret it as threatening. This threat perception causes them to avoid those activities in order to avoid pain. The fear-avoidance behaviour becomes the precursor of further strengthening of fears. A circular, never-ending chain is thus formed.

Hypervigilance is yet another manifestation of fear. Chronic pain can make a person hypervigilant to any cue that increases the pain. In fact, the treatment process quite often gets disrupted because the hypervigilant and fearful patient may not be willing to comply with the exercise regimen chalked out by their doctor or physiotherapist as we saw in Mrs Annu's case in chapter 3.

Loneliness and isolation: Acute pain is usually well-understood, empathized with and given focused attention by family and friends of the patients. However, in chronic pain, due to the very chronicity of pain, sympathy gradually wanes as other aspects of daily living take precedence, leaving little room for spending quality time with the patient. Chronic pain patients are often left to themselves and this makes them feel isolated and lonely as in the case of Mrs Indu, discussed at the beginning of this chapter.

Sometimes this isolation is self-created, but most often it happens due to the exigencies of one's very existence. In some conditions, like rheumatoid arthritis, fear-avoidance may cause the sufferer to shy away from being in close proximity to people, for fear of accidental or a careless touch that could cause pain (hypervigilance). One such patient confided smilingly to me that she never shook hands with anyone, as a vigorous handshake would leave her with pain for several days. Lack of touch, warmth related to touch, emotional comfort derived from touch could all be missing from a chronic patient's life. Many patients complain of not being understood, not being heard out patiently and, often, not being shown empathy.

Physical and emotional fatigue: Chronic pain can engender both physical and emotional fatigue. The body has a natural mechanism to heal on its own, but in a chronic pain patient, pain as well as fear of pain quite often restricts free movement of the body and more effort is required to redeploy the body in any kind of activity. This often results in physical fatigue.

Worry or negative emotions like anger, hatred and guilt all consume mental energy that leaves the person mentally and emotionally exhausted. Brooding over an endless list of problems such as ways and means to get better, possible treatment options, fear of disability, financial burdens and even difficult interpersonal relationships can plunge an already tired and yet-to-recover body into weariness. Insomnia, disturbed sleep and non-refreshed sleep are other sources aggravating fatigue.

Impact of pain on other functions

Insomnia: Insomnia is a sleep disorder that is present in nearly all patients of chronic pain. Sleep is a behaviourally regulated drive that maintains physical and mental homeostasis in the body and is very much essential for the well-being of both the body and the mind. Chronic pain and sleep have a reciprocal, bidirectional relationship.

Being in constant pain can affect sleep at night and disturbed sleep can increase pain the next day by lowering the threshold for pain. This leaves the patient perpetually in a state of exhaustion and fatigue. In fact, sleep disorders may be present in 67 to 88 per cent of patients with chronic pain.[8] On the other hand, it has also been observed that nearly 50 per cent of patients with insomnia have chronic pain.[9] Fibromyalgia—with its non-restorative sleep pattern, leaving sufferers unrefreshed the next morning—is the best example of this relationship.

It is interesting to know that regulation of both sleep and pain occurs in certain areas of the brain that are common to both (chapter two). In a recent study of healthy volunteers, it was shown that sleep-deprived persons had increased sensitivity to painful stimuli.[10] Functional MRI done in these persons showed increased activity in the somatosensory area of the brain that is responsible for discrimination of pain. Simultaneously, those areas in the brain that decrease pain by releasing a neurochemical called dopamine, showed less than normal activity. According to Matthew Walker, the senior author of the study, 'Sleep loss not only amplifies the pain-sensing regions in the brain, but blocks the natural analgesia centres, too.' Another area of the brain, the hypothalamus, helps in regulating both pain and sleep. This area of the brain is high in the neurochemical GABA, which is one of the inhibitory neurotransmitters of pain as well as necessary for sleep. So we see that multiple areas of the brain are involved in the experience of pain-related sleep disturbances.

Thus, in a way, sleep is part of the body's own natural analgesic mechanism. Knowing the close relationship between chronic pain and sleep is important in the management of pain, and it is necessary for sleep disturbances to also be dealt with in order to relieve pain.

Sexual difficulties: One of the side-effects of chronic pain is sexual difficulty. Pain may not only be a reason for decreased sexual pleasure but may also be a deterrent for sexual activity because of increase in pain on sexual physicality. Another valid reason for reduced libido may be mood disturbance, like depression, which is usually associated with pain. Stress, which is a natural fallout of chronic pain, is yet an added reason for poor sexual desire and performance. In addition, some medicines used to treat chronic pain itself can affect the libido.

Lowered self-esteem: The emotional and physical difficulties, as mentioned above, that impact a chronic pain patient naturally lower their self-esteem. Self-esteem is a person's sense of self-worth or self-appreciation. This involves belief and appraisal of oneself, physically, emotionally and behaviourally. Nathaniel Branden defined self-esteem as having two interrelated facets—that of a sense of personal efficacy and a sense of personal worth. A combination of these factors gives a person self-confidence and self-respect.[11]

Most persons cherish their independence to walk, work, indulge in desirable activities and interact. Chronic pain tends to *limit* or *alter* the freedom to perform such tasks. A fair number of people with chronic pain have to take help from others for everyday mundane activities like dressing, eating or walking. This dependency could be irksome and, for some, even demeaning. Other distressing factors that could adversely affect the self-esteem of a person in chronic pain are physical deformity, abnormalities in gait or a paralysed limb resulting in movement difficulty.

When self-esteem is low, the person is very likely to feel unloved, lack confidence, have feelings of inadequacy and be inclined to regard self in a negative light. They may be alert to signs of slighting and any delay in providing care could be construed as rejection. Many patients may feel so obligated that they would not ask for anything for fear of further burdening their loved ones. People with low self-esteem also think that they do not deserve any extra love and care. Self-esteem is not a stable characteristic and is prone to fluctuations with changed situations, but as long as it remains low, it negatively impacts the well-being of the person.

Let us now go back to the case of Mrs Indu mentioned at the beginning of the chapter and assess her from the psychological point of view. Chronic pain had played havoc with her psyche as well as her relationships. Since she was immobile and now dependent on her son and daughter-in-law for everyday needs, it added to her feelings of shame and helplessness. She stopped demanding their companionship and stopped complaining of loneliness.

She was clinically depressed when we met her in the hospital, with clear symptoms of low mood, anhedonia (inability to enjoy previously enjoyable activities), helplessness, hopelessness and worthlessness, excessive guilt feelings of being a burden on her son and daughter-in-law and even wished she were dead.

She had sleep disturbance, too, the reason being partly pain, partly stress and depression, and partly uncontrolled diabetes that necessitated frequent nocturnal urination. Sleep disturbance, in turn, was impacting the functioning of her body and mind. The interplay of both bodily and emotional attributes had become the perpetuating and maintaining factors for the chronicity of her pain.

Developing a sick role: One of the most impactful psychological after-effects of chronic pain is development of a sick role. Sick role, as defined by Talcott Parsons, was the society's sanction of 'behaviour of' and 'behaviour towards' a person considered sick/ill by the society.[12] Parson gave two rights and two responsibilities to a sick person. The two rights were (i) not to be blamed for being sick; (ii) not be held responsible for being unable to perform one's routine duties like vocation, occupation, school and household chores. The two responsibilities attributed to the sick person were (i) to make recovery a priority; (ii) to seek help if so required, instead of adopting a sick role.

Later, these rights and responsibilities given by Parsons were considered as being inadequate and Suchman (1965)[13,14] described development of sick role as a process. He gave five distinct stages that lead to such illness behaviour.

a. *The first stage*: is characterized as the *symptom experience*, where the patient feels physical pain and discomfort that becomes associated with an emotional response. An understanding then accrues that there is a possibility of disruption of one's occupational, personal and social functioning.

b. *The second stage*: is typified by the *assumption of the sick role*, when it dawns on the patient about the seriousness of the illness. This leads gradually to relinquishing of the active roles that the person had been playing till then, with transition occurring from being an active member to a sick member of the society.

c. *The third stage*: is distinguished by actively *seeking medical help*. Five '*social triggers*' have been identified that influence the decision for seeking medical aid. The realization that (i) illness is interfering with vocational and professional life, (ii) with social and personal life, (iii) crisis in interpersonal relationships, (iv) pressure from family and friends, (v) 'temporalizing', i.e., giving self a time frame to become better on one's own. These social triggers take into account the patient's background, age, gender, race, ethnicity and social class. Their importance lies in the findings that women (more than men) and married men (more than unmarried men) seek treatment for illness.

d. *The fourth stage*: is exemplified by the emerging *dependent role* and fears of the patient. It addresses issues like cognitive and physical decline, loss of independence, unwelcome bodily changes and loss of key social roles. Ailing persons get more attention, affection, care and exemption from taking responsibilities. All these lead to the development of '*secondary gains*'. Sometimes, secondary gains are visible even after recovery, as seen in persons who complain of pain when expected to help others or those who perform only those tasks that are pleasurable to them.
   e. *The fifth stage*: involves *rehabilitation*. Once patients reach this stage, they modify and change their lifestyles and make adjustments to the decline in physical, mental and social situations. These adjustments depend also upon the attitude and previous adjustments within the family, couple relationship, cohesiveness and dynamics between the family members.

Impact within the family

Couple relationship: Chronic pain in one member can impact the entire family, but the relationship that gets affected the most is the couple's bond. Most marriages start with wellness and good health. However, when one partner develops chronic pain there are obvious as well as subtle changes in the relationship. Initially, then subsequently, the healthier partner may have to don the mantle of responsibilities of both, which may bring changes in their equation with each other. This is likely to be stressful for the healthier partner. A lot depends upon how the healthier partner reacts to changes in life and his/her ability to cope with the situation. An impatient and easily perturbed healthier partner may handle even simple challenges with strain.

The lifestyle of the healthier partner gets altered not only by the extra amount of work that inadvertently falls into their lap, but also by other factors such as: having to perhaps be both father and mother to the children; coping with financial difficulties; taking care of medical appointments; poor sexual satisfaction; their own health and exercise regimen; lack of leisure activities and socialization; and coping with an emotionally disturbed spouse.

Most people are ill-prepared for the sudden contingency of medical demands and may have difficulty in shifting gears and realigning their lives. Couples and families that have a cohesive relationship are better able to organize themselves to the demands placed upon them, though one should never demean or diminish the struggle they go through. The reverse is equally true. Couples with already frayed or disjointed relationships face more difficulties, which may even lead to expressed emotions and marital dysfunctionality or even discord and separation.

Change in interpersonal relations in the family: Ultimately, it is the family that has to invariably rally around any permanent changes that are likely to happen when one member is chronically ill or disabled. Certain fundamental characteristics of the family that could help tide over—or at least those characteristics that assist to maintain a decorum of dealing with difficulties—are emotional, social, financial and economic stability, perception of control, easy transition of roles and conflict-free role reversals. These will depend upon family cohesiveness, personalities of the family members and their own innate ability to cope with stress. A blend of the above factors ensures the well-being and good care of the patient, and some semblance of normalcy and even happiness amongst family members may be seen despite the troubles they are going through.

Physical and Psychological Impact of Chronic Pain

Role reversal (becoming a patient) is especially difficult for those who are insecure and vulnerable and who tend to take offence at even trivial issues as they find themselves losing their prestige and stature in the house. The respect and deference that they may have once commanded may no longer be theirs. Such persons in all likelihood would be problematical and uncooperative with the family and difficult to treat as well.

The effect on caregivers—stress, burnout and expressed emotions: While discussing the psychological impact of chronic pain on the sufferer, let us not forget the impact it has on the caregiver, be it the spouse or the family. The amount of time, effort and commitment that the caregivers need to give to a chronic pain patient would, in most likelihood, deplete their physical capacity, sap them emotionally and exhaust them mentally. Prolonged caregiving often leads to *burnout*. Burnout happens when the caregiver shows signs of depression, anxiety, irritability, feels run down and chronically fatigued.

Caregivers are often unable to sleep soundly and get up enervated in the morning. They tend to overreact to minor situations and have exaggerated reactions in case new health issues crop up in the patient. Promising outcomes usually keep the caregiver motivated and enthusiastic about caregiving. But when the outcome is bleak and they know that the situation may only partially improve or not at all, the eagerness, keenness and interest in caregiving wanes.

In extreme situations, one may find the caregiver not being able to take care of self. There may be an 'either-or' situation where the needs of the chronic pain patient may take a precedence over one's own needs. In such situations, there is a likelihood of developing *caregiver stress syndrome*. Here the caregiver starts to neglect self to care for the chronically ill patient, resulting in the deterioration of their own physical and mental health. A caregiver's overall health would be dependent on such factors like the amount of time and effort required for caregiving, their own age and health status, relationship with the patient, as well as the gender (as nursing mostly falls in the lap of women).

Some key factors also could be related to the patient such as the patient's behavioural problems, cognitive well-being and degree of functional disabilities. The constant and relentless pressure on the caregiver could change their attitude from being positive and caring, to negative and indifferent and, at times, even to active hostility. This is especially true for caregivers of patients with terminal cancer and in pain, as seen in the case discussed below.

Expressed emotions by family: Nursing by a family member of a patient with chronic pain and, very often, disability, is different from professional nursing—as one's emotions, relationships and expectations are involved. Expressed emotions indicate the intensity of expression of emotions within the family, ranging from high to low and positive (care and concern) to negative (hostile and angry). Negative expressed emotions can be in the form of criticism, open hostility and emotional over-involvement.

In emotional over-involvement, one sees over-protectiveness and self-sacrificing behaviours amongst family members. Criticism of the patient, by the family, can be in the form of disparate comments, disbelieving them and not acknowledging the efforts made as good enough to get better. Hostility is overt criticism or rejection of the patient and is expressed by making negative statements, blaming the patient, displaying uncaring attitude and being either unhelpful or grudgingly helpful.

Some expressed emotion statements may be such as 'he/she is not trying enough', 'so much is being done but he/she does not cooperate', 'he/she does not realize how much we are concerned' or 'how much we are sacrificing for him/her', 'our lives are also on hold' and so on. These behaviours or expressed emotions by the caregiver can have a detrimental effect on the psyche of the patient, arousing guilt, anger, resentment, stubbornness or, in worst cases, even aggression. Such expressed emotions become a two-way process with neither the patient nor the family being mentally well. Needless to say, the higher the expressed emotions in the family, the worse the prognosis.

On the other hand, positive, encouraging and appreciative remarks motivate the patient to try their best to improve. Emotional warmth, empathy and an understanding family, which gives space even for their sad moods, stimulates and persuades the patient to keep trying to improve. Thus, the role of the family members, their attitudes, ability to cope with disability and family cohesiveness are all crucial factors for the outcome of the treatment.

Dr Yash is a 76-year-old doctor who had been suffering from throat cancer for the last two-and-a-half years. He had been given all possible medical treatment and was operated on several times for the same. Ultimately his larynx, or the voice box, was removed and he lost his voice permanently.

The radiation therapy, which was done subsequently for the recurrence of cancer, had caused pain and stiffness in his throat and had also made swallowing of food difficult and painful. An electrolarynx implantation for restoration of his voice was planned, but could not be carried out as he was not fit enough for the surgery. He also suffered from memory loss because of previous episodes of mild strokes. His feeding was only blended food given through a Ryles tube inserted into the stomach through the nose. Besides, there was a long list of medicines to be given too. All this had to be done meticulously according to the doctors' advice.

The chief caregiver was his wife and she had to guess his needs and decipher his written scrawls. This only added to her burden of caregiving. Let us quote one such instance, where she—a caring, loving and affectionate wife—was slowly becoming impatient and angry with her ailing husband who was also suffering from chronic pain. One of the side effects of chemotherapy drugs is constant thirst due to dehydration, and so Dr Yash would continuously demand water to drink. This naturally increased his frequency of urination. Since he had had several prior falls and had even injured himself, every visit to the washroom meant as many awakenings in the night for his wife.

A physically tired, sleep deprived lady, distraught with the fear of losing her beloved husband, was slowly becoming a bitter, irritable, short-tempered and sharp-tongued person. She would often scold him, which made the patient feel guilty and depressed. Since he was handicapped due to his inability to speak, he would often scrawl the word 'sorry' or fold his hands asking for forgiveness. This made his wife more miserable and she would be angry with herself for saying such harsh words to him, knowing full well that his life span was limited. It was a no-win situation for both the patient and the caregiver. Nevertheless, such is the plight of a caregiver and a chronically ill patient.

However, every caregiver is not so distressed. There are some positive effects of caregiving, too. Some rewards of caregiving could be an increased sense of competence, development of ability to cope with situations, appreciation of life, personal growth and enhanced self-esteem and, most importantly, the relationship between the patient and caregiver getting augmented with warmth and closeness.[15]

A 65-year-old workaholic businessman, Raghav, met with an accident that left him with a couple of broken ribs and fracture in his right thigh. He underwent surgery for his thigh fracture. Despite physiotherapy and regular exercises, he was in constant pain and could only limp around with support.

His wife, a homemaker, had always been patient and supportive, not only during this illness but even prior to that, as his work schedule was always demanding. In fact, she had virtually brought up her three children single-handedly and had never complained of lack of attention from her husband. Even when people jokingly questioned her about his apparent lack of concern for her, she always supported her husband saying that he worked hard for them and should not be accused of neglecting his family.

When she saw her husband suffering pain and disability after the accident, she delegated the running of the business to her sons and the running of the house to her daughters-in-law. She moved with her husband into another smaller house nearby, where she could devotedly look after him. She helped him with his exercises, accompanied him for walks, ensured his meals were on time and cooked high-protein nutritious food for him.

She was indeed busier now than ever before, but she was cherishing the time spent alone with him, which had never happened earlier. Despite the pain the gentleman was suffering, the couple actually said that they had at last found each other after almost thirty-five years of marriage.

Thus, caregiving for a chronically ill person need not always be burdensome, it can at times be rewarding and enriching for the patient and the caregiver.

Social relationships: For chronic pain patients, social relations often take a backseat. This, of course, depends upon the severity of the disability and degree of residual mobility. Those who have minimal pain and can sustain the rigours of social life, tend to preserve their social network. Social isolation is not a happy condition to be in. It need not necessarily be intentional, but may stem from the patient's own thoughts or fears. Chronic pain patients feel that their pain and disability may not be understood by others and perhaps even carry the fear of being disbelieved, laughed at, shamed, ostracized or simply rejected. Very often, instead of others snubbing them, the patient tends to rebuff others by secluding themselves. Apart from loneliness, such seclusion does not help in taking one's mind off pain, as social interaction is a good form of distraction, aids in the feeling of connectedness and gives the comfort of togetherness.

Work, Employment and Economic Stress

Chronic pain impacts employability. Most employers prefer able-bodied, efficient, dependable and reliable employees. A chronic pain patient may be compelled to often call in sick, leading to absenteeism or irregular appearance at office. They could perhaps not be able to fulfil their job requirements, meet deadlines or accomplish the desired outcome of job expectations. This often puts the patient in a dilemma about disclosure of their pain condition.

Disclosure is a double-edged sword. The patient, who discloses to the employer about their condition, has expectations of some work-related concessions or compensations such as overlooking absenteeism and even shoddy work. They may also expect being eased into a lesser stressful job profile without any financial implications. On the other hand, the employer is faced with considerations of incomplete work, less efficiency, unnecessary resentment amongst other employees and many other factors. Thus, generally employers feel hesitant to keep persons with chronic pain on their payroll.

Other equally important factors that influence the employability of chronic pain patients is their age, education and job status.

Frequently, it has been seen that the older the individual and lesser the education, the more their vulnerability to job loss and unemployment. Their stress is likely to be higher as well because lack of education would not allow them to shift to an altogether different type of work. People who do manual (blue collar) jobs have greater susceptibility to unemployment due to chronic pain. Lack of employment or lower income, cost of medical treatment, number of dependents, lack of savings and many such factors can contribute to economic stress for the patient.

However, an empathetic employer can ease and adjust the stress of the pain-ridden person by re-deployment or providing opportunity to work from home or allowing a phased return to work, starting with the least burdensome work. A gainfully employed person is more motivated to get better, with fewer psychological issues. Let me give an example to illustrate this point.

A 34-year-old man, Vinay, who worked as a supervisor in the Delhi Metro Rail Corporation, was suffering from chronic back pain. He was finding it difficult to do his work as it involved a lot of physical activity and climbing up and down ramps. He was the sole breadwinner of his family, which comprised his elderly parents, wife and two small children who lived in his hometown. However, his immediate supervisor was a considerate boss. He advised Vinay to first priotize proper treatment for his back pain and reassured him of his place in the organization post his return. And that is what Vinay did. After taking three months off for his pain management treatment, he rejoined work as a happier man who could carry out his duties effectively without much pain.

We have seen how nearly every aspect of a person's life gets affected due to chronic pain. This rippling effect casts a shadow even on the lives of their caregivers and other persons who are closely associated with them. It is, therefore, important, nay imperative, that the patient is provided with treatment at the earliest and in a holistic manner. But before the actual management of chronic pain is started, a comprehensive assessment of pain has to be done, along with an assessment of the level of dysfunctionality and disability. This requires a detailed assessment of physical, psychological and social factors contributing to chronic pain and whether these are assets or impediments to the management of pain. The next chapter deals with the issue of assessment of chronic pain.

6

Assessment in Chronic Pain

We have understood chronic pain from a biopsychosocial perspective. We have seen that when the pain becomes chronic, the cognitive (thoughts) and affective (emotions) inputs gain precedence over the sensory inputs in creating pain perceptions. Therefore, when a patient presents with chronic pain, just a physical assessment would be incomplete as the very definition of pain states that it is both an unpleasant physical and emotional experience. By merely assessing the physical component, neither would we arrive at the right diagnosis, nor would our treatment be appropriate. A comprehensive pain assessment would, therefore, entail assessment of the physical, functional and psychosocial components contributing to chronic pain so that an appropriate treatment regime can be charted out to address all the relevant issues.

Taking a Patient's History

Taking a patient's history is crucial for the assessment of pain, as it tells the story of the sufferer. For this, first and foremost, the treating doctor needs to gain the trust of, and develop a rapport with, both the patient and the caregiver. Only then will they confide their problems, both physical as well as psychological, that would provide a clue to the diagnosis. Otherwise—to anyone taking a cursory history, or to an impatient clinician be it a pain specialist, a clinical psychologist, or a physiotherapist—they will not normally divulge subtle details.

Besides the history of pain, it is also important to take family and occupation history, drug and medication history and history of comorbidities. Family history could provide a clue to whether the pain has a genetic predisposition; occupation history may reveal whether any work-related factors could be contributory. This is followed by mental status examination to obtain a comprehensive cross-sectional description of the patient's mental state. All this requires careful and sensitive handling so that the patient cooperates with the initial assessment and later adheres to the treatment being offered.

Assessing patients with acute pain, such as pain after an injury or surgery, is usually straightforward and can be done with various tools that can assess the intensity or severity of pain. Chronic pain, on the other hand, which has a history of lasting more than three months and sometimes even years, in all likelihood would have affected the functioning of the patient, may have caused disability and would have had psychological repercussions as well. Assessment of such patients is, therefore, more complicated, complex and challenging as—besides pain, which itself can be variegated—the functional status, psychological and social status have to be assessed.

Let us discuss these factors one by one.

Assessment of Pain

A useful mnemonic for assessment of pain is PQRST.

P—provoking and alleviating factors. Those factors that aggravate the pain and those that relieve it.

Q—quality of pain, whether it is pricking, burning, shooting, gnawing, electric current-like, etc.

R—radiation of pain to other sites in the body. For e.g., low back pain can radiate to the legs, shoulder pain can radiate to the head, pain from the appendix can radiate to the umbilicus (belly button), etc.

S—site (location) and severity of pain.

T—temporal nature of pain: does it increase or decrease during the day or has it increased or decreased over time.

Each of the parameters mentioned above can provide a clue to the possible diagnosis.

Besides these, one also has to assess the type of pain and from where it is primarily originating. For example, it could be due to tissue damage, as with chronic inflammation (nociceptive), or a disease of the nervous system (neuropathic), or from muscles and its coverings or fascia (myofascial), etc. Many a time, it could be due to a combination of factors.

Pain Assessment Tools

The gold standard of measurement of pain is always the patient's own report of his or her pain or, in other words, 'self-report'. To reiterate Margo McCaferry's simple definition of pain, 'It is whatever the experiencing patient says it is, existing whenever and wherever the patient says it does.'[1] The pain specialist should believe what the patient says about the intensity of pain. Even in patients with dementia or Alzheimer's disease, irrespective of the cognitive state of the patient, the first step is always to ask the patient about their pain. Only, thereafter, is the caregiver questioned.

To facilitate more objective measurement of pain, there are well-validated pain assessment tools that help not only in assessing the severity of pain, but can track the response of pain to treatment over time. These pain assessment tools can be unidimensional which means that only one dimension of pain is measured, namely the severity of pain. Then there are multidimensional tools that are more descriptive and can assess the overall impact pain has on the physical, psychological and social health of the person. Besides, there are tools to assess whether the pain is neuropathic in nature.

Let us discuss these individually.

Unidimensional tools

These are the most commonly used tools to measure the intensity of pain, the main advantage being its simplicity. In the Numerical Rating Scale (NRS), the patient is asked to quantify pain on a scale, where 0 is no pain and 10 is worst imaginable pain. In the Visual Analogue Scale (VAS),[2] the patient marks the severity of pain on a straight line marked from 0 to 10, where 0 indicates no pain and 10 the most severe pain. A body map may also be provided where the exact location and radiation of pain, if present can be pinpointed by the patient.

The Wong-Baker FACES Pain Rating Scale[3] is used mostly for children and for some adults who cannot categorize their pain on the scales mentioned above, either because of cognitive difficulty or language barrier or if they are not literate. The scale depicts six faces with different expressions, starting from smiling face to a crying face—the smiling face signifies no pain and the crying face indicates severe pain. The appropriate image is then selected to match with the patients' expression (be it a child or an adult).

The FLACC scale[4] is yet another scale used mainly for infants depending on the premise that the body language of the baby indicates the degree of pain. 'FLACC' is a mnemonic for Face, Legs, Activity, Cry and Consolability. These indices are used to assess the level of pain in the infant.

Multidimensional scales

These are more complex measuring tools for pain, which not only assess the severity of pain but also the effect pain has on the patient's emotions, functionality as well as social health. In other words, multidimensional scales can assess pain in a truly holistic manner. The most commonly used multidimensional scales are McGill's Pain Questionnaire (MPQ),[5] and Brief Pain Inventory.[6] The MPQ is a three-dimensional questionnaire that can assess the sensory, emotional and the evaluative aspects of pain. The Brief Pain Inventory assesses the intensity of pain and the effect pain has on the activities of the patient.

West Haven Yale Multidimensional Pain Inventory (WHYMPI)[7]

This is a 52-item self-administered rating scale. The scale measures all the three components, namely cognitions, affect and behaviour of the patient. It has three major domains that subsume twelve sub-scales. The three domains are pain experience, significant others response to pain experience and patient's participation in daily activities. The first domain of pain experience captures the patient's perceived interference in daily activities, pain severity, control over pain, perceived support from significant others and emotional response to pain. The second domain of Significant Others Response to Pain is seen by the perception of patient's perceived frequencies of punishing, solicitous and distracting responses. The third domain of Participation in Daily Activities measures the ability to perform household chores, outdoor activities, social activities and those activities that are away from home.

As mentioned earlier, it is important to differentiate nociceptive from neuropathic pain. Tools that assess neuropathic pain take into account symptoms and signs that are commonly seen as burning pain, tingling and abnormal sensations, pain on touch, exaggerated response to a painful stimulus, etc. Some commonly used questionnaires to assess neuropathic pain are the Leeds Assessment of Neuropathic Symptoms and Signs (LANSS),[8] Douleur Neuropathique (DN4)[9] and pain DETECT.[10]

Psychosocial Assessment

We have already gathered the importance of psychological factors in the perception of pain. Psychological assessment is to determine those psychosocial factors that are causing, maintaining and acting as barriers in regaining, as far as possible, the previous level of well-being of the person. Disturbances in mood and cognitions that do not amount to classified psychiatric disorders, but have a bearing on the adaptation, adjustment, development of disability and the functionality (social, occupational and personal) of the person, need to be tapped as well.

Psychosocial assessment includes assessment of comorbid symptoms, affective vulnerability, beliefs and attitudes and social/environmental factors.[11] Let us now evaluate each in a little more detail.

Comorbid symptoms

Chronic pain is often accompanied by fatigue, sleep disturbances, impairment in physical functioning and difficulty in concentration and memory, which also includes cognitive functioning. The following tests can be used to measure these functions.

Multiple Abilities Symptom Questionnaire (MASQ):[12] is a 38-item questionnaire that measures cognitive impairment in the domains of language, visuo-perception, verbal memory, visual memory and attention. It is a self-reported questionnaire and picks up cognitive difficulty like fibro fog, or brain fog, as typically seen in patients with fibromyalgia.

Multidimensional Fatigue Inventory (MFI):[13] is a 20-item rating scale used for measuring five dimensions of fatigue: general fatigue, physical fatigue, reduced motivation, reduced activity and mental fatigue. It is a self-reported inventory that ranges from 'Yes, that is true' to 'No, that is not true'.

Pittsburgh Sleep Quality Index (PSQI):[14] is a questionnaire that has 19 self-rated questions and 5 questions rated by the bed partner or roommate, provided one is available. Scoring is only done for the 19 self-rated questions. Seven components are interpreted, namely subjective sleep quality, sleep latency, sleep duration, habitual sleep efficiency, sleep disturbances, use of sleep medicines and daytime dysfunctionality. Each component ranges from 0–3 points.

Affective vulnerability

Depression, anxiety, anger dyscontrol and emotional upheaval, as seen in some personality disorders, can coexist with chronic pain and these come under the ambit of affective vulnerability. There are innumerable scales to measure them. Some of the common and frequently used ones are described below.

Beck's Depression Inventory:[15] is a 21-item self-administered rating scale that measures symptoms like low mood, guilt feelings, biological disturbances, fatigue, suicidal ideation and somatic symptoms.

Depression and Anxiety Stress Scale (DASS):[16] is a 42-item scale divided into three sub-sections of depression, anxiety and stress, as the name indicates. Each sub-section has 14 items with numerical rating. Summation of the score gives us the severity of each of the three conditions.

The Center for Epidemiological Studies-Depression (CES-D):[17] is a 20-item self-reported scale that measures symptoms associated with depression in the last six weeks. There are six scales that measure different aspects of depression like depressed mood, feelings of helplessness and hopelessness, guilt feelings and worthlessness, psychomotor retardation, disturbed sleep and loss of appetite.

Beck's Anxiety Inventory:[18] is a 21-item self-administered rating scale that measures various anxiety symptoms like anxious mood, tensions, fears, insomnia, as well as cardiovascular, respiratory, autonomic, gastrointestinal and genitourinary symptoms. This scale, too, is graded as normal, mild, moderate and severe—reflecting the severity of the condition.

Penn's State Worry Questionnaire (PSWQ):[19] is a 16-item self-administered questionnaire that is often paired with other anxiety scales, like Beck's Anxiety Inventory, as it measures the cognitive component of anxiety like catastrophizing. It is a 5-point rating scale that indicates the trait of worry and is helpful in differentiating people with Generalized Anxiety Disorder (GAD) from other anxiety disorders.

State Trait Anxiety Inventory (STAI):[20] is a 20-item self-reported inventory that differentiates between state and trait anxiety. State anxiety is the transient psychological and physiological reaction to a stressful situation, whereas trait anxiety is a personality trait that indicates individual differences in reaction to an adverse situation; STAI measures both the trait and state anxieties.

State Trait Anger Expression Inventory (STAXI):[21] is a 44-item self-administered, 4-point rating scale. There are five independent sub-scales: State Anger, Trait Anger, Anger-in, Anger-out and Anger Control. A summation of scores on three sub-scales—Anger-in, Anger-out and Anger Control—gives the general index of the frequency with which the person expresses anger.

Positive and Negative Affect Scale (PANAS):[22] is a self-reported 5-point rating measure of both the positive and negative affect. There are 20 adjectives—10 of positive affect and 10 of negative affect—describing the mood states. The summation of positive affect scores reflects positive affect state and summation of negative affect scores reflects negative affect state. Lower scores on negative affect scales represent lower levels of negative affect.

Beliefs and attitudes

Beliefs and attitudes play a major role in developing, maintaining and at times acting as barriers in treatment efficacy. It is, therefore, important to gauge a patient's pain-specific beliefs related to curability of pain, onus of responsibility of pain management, clinician's role, family's role, effectiveness and types of treatment available and so on. Other critical beliefs include beliefs about control over one's condition, locus of control, coping options available, ability to utilize the resources and resilience. The most crucial factor is catastrophizing the pain condition, which is linked to poor outcomes. Thus, beliefs and attitudes either help a person to become better or act as a barrier in the treatment programme.

Beliefs in Pain Control Questionnaire (BPCQ):[23] is a 13-item questionnaire that measures the strength of a person's beliefs regarding pain control, which have been sub-divided into three factors, namely belief in personal control (internal factors), belief that powerful others control pain (doctor's interventions/other powers) or belief that pain is controlled by chance (chance events).

Coping Strategies Questionnaire (CSQ):[24] is a 50-item questionnaire that measures an array of cognitive and behavioural coping strategies. There are six cognitive strategies and one behavioural one. These have been clubbed under three factors: coping actively (that comprises re-evaluation of pain perceptions, ignoring perceptions, declared coping); diverting attention and creating distractions (that includes diverting attention and increase in behavioural activity); and catastrophizing and seeking hope.

Pain Self-Efficacy Questionnaire (PSEQ):[25] is a 10-item questionnaire that taps the patient's confidence in his/her ability to perform activities despite pain. It is a 7-point rating scale, with 0 indicating 'not at all confident' to 6 which is 'completely confident'. The summation of score suggests the self-efficacy of the patient.

Pain Catastrophizing Scale (PCS):[26] is a self-administered 13-item 5-point rating scale. The scale measures three aspects of catastrophizing, namely rumination, magnification and helplessness in management of pain.

Social interactions and environmental factors

Conducive social interactions and environment play a vital role in the effectiveness of the treatment programme. It is, therefore, important to assess the role of the family, caregivers and significant persons in the patient's life. Other stressors—such as job dissatisfaction, unhappy married life or financial difficulties—also need to be known, so that overall understanding of the patient is better.

Dyadic Adjustment Scale (DAS):[27] is a 32-item self-administered scale. It measures a person's perception of the relationship with their intimate partner. It portrays the parameters of consensus, satisfaction, cohesion and affection between partners.

There are innumerable scales that measure relationship satisfaction between couples and within family. Some commonly used ones are Marital Satisfaction Scale, Dyadic Communication Scale, Family Adjustment Scale and Family Conflict Assessment, among many others. Relationship tests are only required to be administered if conflictual relationship is becoming a reason for the patient to be stressed, unhappy, depressed or anxious, thereby inadvertently increasing pain experience.

Other requisite tests for psychological assessment are discussed briefly below.

Assessment of personality

As we have already seen in the previous chapters, some types of personality traits and personality types show resilience in the face of adversity, while some tend to succumb. Measuring personality traits helps when the pain patient is taken up for psychotherapy.

Eysenck Personality Questionnaire-Revised (EPQ-R):[28] is a self-administered forced choice ('yes or no') test with 48 items. It measures neuroticism, psychoticism and extroversion and also has a 'Lie' scale. A high score on the Lie scale indicates that the findings of the test are not reliable, as the person may have been faking or giving socially desirable responses. The Neuroticism sub-scale shows the emotional adjustment of the person and high scores on the scale indicates a tendency towards anxiety, depression, worry, fears, anger, guilt and loneliness. Neuroticism tendencies are normally high in persons who develop chronic pain. The Psychoticism sub-scale measures traits of dominance-leadership, dominance-submission, lack of superego (conscience) and sensation-seeking behaviour. The Extroversion sub-scale categorizes the person as being either an introvert or an extrovert. The EPQ-R is a short test that requires about ten minutes to complete it.

Rotter's Locus of Control Scale (LOC):[29] is a 29-item scale in which there are six buffer items that are not scored. It is a forced choice scale, with higher scores indicating external locus of control and lower scores indicating internal locus of control. It measures the personality characteristic of perceived control, which is a stable trait and does not vary with mood or situations. A person with internal locus of control would have higher self-esteem, confidence in own abilities, more coping options and higher self-mastery.

Though these tests are easy to administer and quick to score, they have a major limitation in terms of response set. Response set is a tendency to mark the same response to all items irrespective of the content of the question. For example, a patient may mark 0 (minimum score) or 3 (maximum score) on nearly all the test items. This gives a skewed image of the presence of a disorder, which may be different from reality.

Assessment Using Projective Tests: Projective tests are so designed that the response of a person to an ambiguous stimulus reveals the hidden emotions and conflicts that may not be otherwise apparent. Projective tests are valuable as there is no response set or response bias, thus reducing fake or socially desirable responses, are not over-dependent on verbal abilities and tap both conscious and unconscious traits of a person. There are five types of projective techniques: Word Association; Completion Tests; Construction Tests; Expression Tests; and Choice or Ordering.

Of the above five techniques, three have been found to be significantly helpful in clinical practice. These are the Completion method (where Sentence Completion Test is used), the Construction method (where the Thematic Apperception Test is used) and the Association method (where the Rorschach Inkblot Test is used). These tests are useful in picking up both personality traits and pathognomonic signs of major psychiatric illnesses.

Sack's Sentence Completion Test (SSCT):[30] is a semi-structured test with 60 incomplete sentences that have to be completed with the first thought that comes to the mind. It measures areas like relationship and attitude towards family, work and colleagues, self-concept and heterosexual relationships. Any hidden conflicts and relationship disturbances can also be gleaned from the test.

Thematic Apperception Test (TAT):[31] is based on the assumption that the narratives built around an ambiguous picture card, reflect underlying motives, needs, conflicts and the manner in which the social world is perceived. The story needs to incorporate the past happenings, current scenario and the outcome of the narrated event. The basic assumption of TAT is that the story written or told by the patient actually depicts the disposition and significant incidents from the life of the storyteller. While evaluating the story, the characters drawn on the card, as well as additional characters not in the card, are noted because they give relevant information about the patient.

Rorschach Inkblot Test:[32] 10 ambiguous cards are shown to the person being tested and the responses are recorded verbatim. The responses provide data about the person's thoughts, emotions, needs, motives, conflicts, inner tensions and personal and interpersonal perceptions. This test is useful for eliciting personality traits, emotional functioning and majorly for diagnostic purposes. This test also is helpful in picking up 'pathognomonic' signs of mental disorders.

Let us come back to the case of Mrs Annu (chapter 3) who was hypervigilant and had issues related to her family, in particular, her daughter-in-law. She was described as being 'volatile' by the family. A battery of tests was administered which evaluated the physical, psychological and social aspects of pain. These included Numerical Rating Score (NRS), Brief Pain Inventory (BPI), Eysenck Personality

Questionnaire-Revised (EPQ-R), Depression and Anxiety Stress Scale (DASS), Pain Catastrophizing Scale (PCS), Sack's Sentence Completion Test (SSCT) and Thematic Apperception Test (TAT).

On EPQ-R she showed an extremely high score on neuroticism, suggesting proneness for anxiety, worry, fears, anger and depression. On PCS, she had many catastrophizing thoughts. 'I worry all the time about whether the pain will end'; 'I become afraid that the pain will get worse'; 'I can't seem to keep it out of my mind'; 'I wonder whether something serious may happen', were some of them.

The SSCT and TAT both depicted her anger, nay rage, towards her daughter-in-law. In several TAT stories she had depicted the protagonist as being helpless in alleviating the pain, inability to deal with an errant daughter-in-law, feeling lonely and unloved, anger towards husband for not giving her importance in her own house, fear of losing her son to his wife and above all being disabled for the rest of her life. The DASS had indicated elevated scores on all the three subtests (depression, anxiety and stress). Anxiety, anger, depression and fears were predominantly present on several tests, especially SSCT and TAT.

These findings helped in pinpointing the behaviours and thoughts that needed rectification. It also brought forth the need for family intervention to ease out the dysfunctionality within the family. The test findings gave the patient an insight into her own behaviour and thoughts, and how it was affecting her emotionally, physically and mentally.

Pain Assessment in the Elderly with or without Dementia

This can be difficult for various reasons, which include physical, psychological and intellectual reasons. Impairment in hearing and decreased vision are some of the physical causes that may pose a barrier for assessment of pain in elderly people. Many of them may have difficulty communicating as well, others may be stoic about their pain not wanting to complain about it. Still others believe that pain is an integral part of ageing and has to be accepted as a part of life. It was seen in rural Nepal, and among the Aborginal peoples in Australia, that a substantial number of men and women suffered from back pain but never sought treatment even when offered, as they firmly believed that pain was part of the ageing process and cannot be treated.[33]

Assessment of pain in dementia

There are many elderly people who have dementia or cognitive impairment and are not be able to communicate their pain. In such patients, the assessment of pain is often inadequate and pain is often undertreated as it may not even be recognized. Some tips for assessing pain in patients with dementia are as follows:

- Firstly, directly ask the patient about their pain. This may or may not be forthcoming due to their underlying cognitive problems.
- Secondly, we can question their caregivers about the functionality of the patient and whether there are problems in their daily activities suggestive of pain interfering with it.
- Thirdly, we can look for non-verbal cues or implicit behavioural changes in the patient, which could indicate they are having pain such as grimacing, knitted brows, hesitation or even refusal to move about and do their normal activities. There could be more explicit behaviours like moaning or groaning, cursing, agitation or restlessness. Many may show signs of irritation, anger, anxiety or depression.
- Lastly, in patients with severe cognitive impairment, the Pain Assessment in Advanced Dementia (PAINAD)[34] is a useful scale to measure pain.

Barriers to Pain Assessment

These could be broadly classified as patient barriers, professional barriers and system barriers. Some patient barriers to pain assessment include reluctance of patients to report pain fearing that they may be having a serious underlying disease or fearing the side effects of the treatment for pain. Some fear that they may be distracting their primary doctor from treating the underlying cause of pain, such as cancer. Most chronic pain patients are hypersensitive, easily upset and defensive when asked questions about their pain. Many feel that they are not being believed, criticized or, worse, considered to be imparting falsehoods especially when the family gives a contradictory history.

Another patient barrier is an inability to communicate the nature and intensity of pain, which is especially seen in elderly people with cognitive impairment and in small children. Ethnicity and culture can be a patient barrier, especially when the administrator of tests has their own set of stereotypes and prejudices.

There could be professional barriers for proper assessment of pain, the most important one being a common tendency among clinicians to treat the 'disease' rather than treating the 'person'. Treating the 'person' would mean treating pain in its totality, by addressing the physical, psychological and social aspects. Failure to establish a rapport, lack of empathy or plain indifference are some barriers in getting a proper history to aid assessment of pain. Patients would be forthcoming in revealing their history only with careful and sensitive handling. Otherwise, many crucial factors that could be contributory to pain may be missed. The physician's lack of knowledge could be yet another barrier for assessment of pain. As the saying goes, 'What the mind does not know, the eye does not see.'

An important system-related barrier to pain assessment is failure to refer the patient to the appropriate healthcare provider—be it the pain specialist, clinical psychologist or physiotherapist—who can do the proper assessment of pain from their perspective as well.

Cultural factors are another set of significant barriers in pain assessment. The relationship and communication between the physician and the patient are of vital importance. Language barriers, culture-based attitudes, prejudices and biases can seriously hinder pain assessment and treatment. A few examples would well illustrate these points. It has been seen that in the West, in countries with predominantly White population, African Americans, Hispanics, Asians and Native Americans are likely to be at significant risk for under treatment of pain.[35]

Some ethnic groups are seen to be uncomfortable discussing bodily issues (including pain) with the doctor, because of modesty. Amongst Japanese patients, it is considered unacceptable to complain about gastrointestinal problems and so they make it a point to never mention having opioid-induced constipation or nausea.[36] Many Asians and Christian African Americans consider pain and suffering as necessary for personal redemption or purification.[37] Hesitancy in communicating their pain could be a barrier for assessment of pain in such patients and it could remain inadequately treated.

Physical Examination

Having taken a detailed history of pain and psychosocial issues, a comprehensive physical examination is conducted. It provides further clues as to the diagnosis of the patient. This could include examination of the site of pain, a general physical examination as well as examination of various related systems. For example, a patient with chronic back pain with sciatica would need an examination of the muscular, nervous and skeletal system to make a conclusive and correct diagnosis.

A case study would help illustrate this point.

A 55-year-old lady presented with low back pain that radiated down to the left leg. The pain was severe and she had difficulty in standing and walking even a few steps. The pain was excruciating and shooting in nature and was associated with tingling and numbness of her left leg.

A neurological examination revealed that she could not walk on her heels and she had a foot drop, i.e., she was not able to raise the front part of her foot. The sensations over her left foot also were diminished. An MRI spine confirmed the diagnosis of a prolapsed intervertebral disc (slipped disc) at lumbar 4-5 level, which was compressing the nerve going to the foot. She needed urgent surgery to remove the offending disc. This highlights the importance of neurological examination in a patient with sciatica.

Similarly, patients with headaches, pain in the neck, pelvic and cancer pain, or for that matter, pain anywhere in the body require a thorough clinical evaluation so that serious underlying problems are ruled out before initiating a holistic pain management.

Investigations

The next step in the assessment of pain is conducting investigations that are relevant for the patient. These include blood tests and radiological investigations and help in further clinching the diagnosis. Most patients who present to the pain specialist have invariably been worked up or relevant information may often be available. Very often there may not be any need to get any further tests done. Nevertheless, a review of these and some repeat tests may be necessary to arrive at a diagnosis.

Some tests that need to be done in patients with chronic pain, besides routine blood tests, are checking the serum vitamin D3, vitamin B12, HbA1C and HLA-B27. In patients with painful diabetic neuropathy, aggressive glycaemic control is essential and serum HbA1C levels is very helpful in this regard. Similarly, in patients with neuropathic pain due to peripheral neuropathy, repleting vitamin B12, if there is a deficiency, can along with other modalities, potentially reverse the pain. As mentioned in chapter five, the incidence of vitamin D3 deficiency is high in our country, and this, too, can predispose to musculoskeletal pains. In fact, the deficiency of vitamin D3 and B12 is so common, it is almost like a silent epidemic. HLA-B27 is another useful screening test in patients with pain originating in the spine to rule out spondyloarthropathy, as in the case of Mrs Yogita discussed in chapter four.

Thus, we see that the assessment of a patient with chronic pain has to be from a biopsychosocial perspective to get a clear and complete picture. This enables the multidisciplinary team to pick up salient and vital clues that needs to be addressed when the patient comes for a pain rehabilitation programme. Let us now see how medical therapy, pain interventions, physical therapy and psychotherapies are used for helping the patient in a holistic manner, so that a multidisciplinary treatment strategy can be implemented.

7

Managing Chronic Pain

Each chronic pain patient has a poignant story that goes a little beyond pain. A mind already grappling with pain has a gamut of varying degrees of physical, emotional and social struggles to be reckoned with. Each story is embellished with fears, suffering and emotional torments related to being misunderstood and not believed, attempts to find cures and not getting better and, ultimately, ruined hopes and dreams. The corollary of all these is anger, frustration, anxiety and distress, which, like pain, become cohorts of chronicity.

These trials and tribulations, emotions and feelings, attitudes and beliefs form, unarguably, the crux of chronic pain. When the focus is myopic with the lens only on physical pain, viewed solely as a biomedical experience and treated with unimodal therapies, we as clinicians, are doing a disservice to a patient suffering from chronic pain. The road to recovery in chronic pain can only happen when we defocus from the body and learn to treat the person in entirety as an 'individual' with many faceted issues.

Allow me to reproduce from a patient, Mrs Ankita's diary, how fibromyalgia pain affected her.

'Let me tell you about my relationship with pain. I was diagnosed with a condition called fibromyalgia around five years back and it continues to be my companion, albeit an unwanted one. To explain the condition to you in simple words, it's when your entire body hurts all the time, even without any sickness or injury. They say that the brain does a little trick with the pain signals and people like us end up experiencing pain far more intensely than others. It's almost like pain is flowing through me as organically as any biological fluid would in my body. Fibromyalgia also causes several other difficulties like fatigue, sleeplessness, concentration and memory problems, depression, anxiety, headaches and so on. So, honestly speaking, there is very little respite.

'It took me a little while to get a grip on my condition. But by then it had almost become like my alter ego with a personality of its own and, ironically, it tightened its grip on me. The nature and intensity of pain would fluctuate daily due to varying reasons—right from the changing weather to change in mood. Nevertheless, it continued being debilitating. With prolonged experience of this condition, my mental and emotional structure started to crumble. I started getting more and more irritable, angry, frustrated, pessimistic and guilt-ridden. My self-worth was at an all-time low. My approach towards life, attitude and behaviour, all got consumed by this monster called Pain.

'But what was interesting was that the more physical pain I was in, the more the psychological pain it caused me. I became increasingly grumpy and unhappy. And the more the psychological pain I had, the more physical trauma I would go through. So any negative emotional episode would cause my pain to grow exponentially. It was as if the stress and the pain were feeding into each other, and it seemed to have become a vicious cycle that I was unable to break.'

One cannot ignore the emotional upheaval that Ankita was facing. Concentrating only on treating her physical pain—without addressing her emotional distress, sleep-related difficulties and low mood—may not have yielded a good outcome. As we see, she also had complaints of memory and concentration difficulty, i.e., brain fog. Being a well-educated person herself and having insight into her own behaviour, she was able to correlate the relationship between physical and psychological pain.

Pain is as old as mankind, and so search for remedies and treatments also dates back to then. In modern science or allopathy, there are definite guidelines and protocols for management of acute pain—such as after surgery, injuries or a simple headache—and, to a large extent, this pain can be relieved. But when pain becomes chronic, not only does the nervous system that transmits and perceives pain undergo a remodelling, but the mind also kicks in, leading to an array of psychological, cognitive and social problems. A body racked with persistent and severe pain invariably wrecks the psyche and emotions.

The combination of all these factors makes management of chronic pain patients a challenge to the healthcare provider. The repeated disappointments of what patients term as 'failed treatment' or not getting satisfactory relief from pain, makes them suspicious and mistrusting of not only the clinicians, but at times even of the treatment modalities. The compliance is mostly poor as the patient feels that since nothing has helped so far, nothing is likely to help in future either. Thus, most continue to be miserable rather than being open to treatment, be it medical or psychological.

Even if they do agree to start treatment, adherence to treatment is always suspect and, as a result, outcomes are likely to be poor. Another not so uncommon occurrence is that they tend to flit from one doctor to another (doctor shopping), in the hope that the next one can provide the magic bullet for their pain. Occasionally, it is the patient who poses the most difficult hurdle and sometimes it is the caregiver (either being over-solicitous or insensitive) who adds on to the existing problem.

As a result, a 'cure' for chronic pain can be very elusive.

Multidisciplinary Rehabilitation

The success of treatment lies in establishing a good clinician–patient rapport and having an effective communication, and that begins as soon as the patient enters the clinician's chamber. Greeting the patient, maintaining eye contact and giving him/her full attention helps to put the person at ease. When the patient communicates about the pain, a sympathetic clinician's open acknowledgment that pain is real, virtually nullifies the debate about the presence or intensity of pain. Listening patiently and being tuned to the emotional overtones, gives an inkling about the mindset of the patient. Any seasoned clinician would know that they have a person for whom treatments have failed, mistrust towards the medical fraternity and medical procedures is high, and the baggage of years of frustration and disappointments cloaks the persona. Such a person has to be dealt with empathy and compassion and given the confidence that a listening ear is present and help is available. To start with, simply reassuring the patient that we would try our utmost to relieve their suffering and being fellow travellers in their journey goes a long way in pain management.

Treatment Goals and Psycho-education

Educating the patient and their family about chronic pain is essential before treatment modalities can be applied. A compliant, trusting and educated patient is the one who is likely to benefit the most. Just as we did with Rahul (chapter one), the concept of chronic pain needs to be made clear to the patient from the outset. It is essential that patients understand the intricacies of chronic pain and how pain can transition from acute to chronic. The goals of alleviating pain—when it is acute and when it becomes chronic—need to be clearly spelt out. The patient also needs to know that despite the best efforts, a 'complete cure' or a fully 'painless' state, as was present initially, may be unrealistic. Rather, realistic goals would encompass returning to acceptable functionality, acknowledging fluctuations in pain states, understanding that pain may also occur for no valid reason and, above all, recognizing how mood and stress levels influences pain perception. Once the goals of therapy are made clear, besides implementing the medical, physical, interventional and psychological therapies, the patient is then directed towards the role of 'self-management'.

Management of Chronic Pain

Since pain is a biopsychosocial phenomenon, the basic tenets for management of chronic pain are medical treatment, treatment of the body, treatment of the mind and management of social issues. Let us discuss these one by one.

Medical Management

This includes medical management with various drugs (pharmacological therapy) and interventional therapies.

Pharmacological therapy for chronic pain

The WHO three-step analgesic ladder was formulated by a team of experts in 1986 with the aim of treating cancer pain, although it is also applicable for acute pain and non-cancer chronic pain.[1] As per this ladder (Fig 7.1), drugs are given depending on the intensity of pain. These include non-opioid drugs such as paracetamol and non-steroidal anti-inflammatory drugs (for step 1 mild pain), weak opioids such as tramadol and tapentadol (for step 2, mild to moderate pain) and strong opioids such as morphine, fentanyl and methadone (for step 3, moderate to severe pain). Besides analgesics, adjuvant drugs are added at each step of the ladder, depending on the presence of other types of coexisting pain and associated symptoms such as anxiety, muscle spasm, insomnia, agitation, etc.

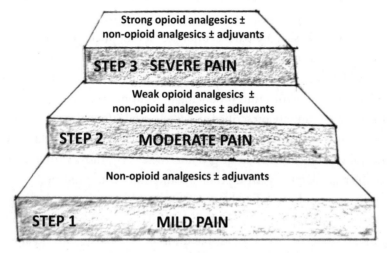

Fig 7.1. The Three-step WHO Analgesic Ladder

Until the WHO analgesic ladder for pain management was introduced more than thirty years ago, pain, cancer pain in particular, was being inadequately treated and people suffered tremendously till their death. This was because potent analgesic drugs such as opioids were not being administered for severe pain, as there was the potential of misuse and addiction. Clinicians, too, were hesitant to prescribe opioids because of the stringent rules and regulations pertaining to their use and misuse. The advent of the WHO analgesic ladder virtually legitimized opioid usage for severe pain, and now nearly 75 per cent of cancer patients are relieved of pain using those drugs in the comfort of their own homes. However, it is wise to use strong opioids such as morphine and its substitutes judiciously for chronic non-cancer pain as there could be misuse and abuse of these drugs leading to fatalities, as has been happening in the West.

Commonly administered analgesics for chronic pain: Medications are invariably the first line of treatment for chronic pain, starting from simple over-the-counter analgesics to more potent drugs (such as opioids). Step 1 analgesics, which are used to treat pain of mild to moderate intensity, are paracetamol (acetaminophen) and the non-steroidal anti-inflammatory drugs (NSAIDs) (Fig 7.1). The latter are called anti-inflammatory drugs because they reduce the release of inflammatory factors, thus producing relief from pain. Paracetamol is the most commonly prescribed and freely available analgesic. Unlike NSAIDs such as ibuprofen and diclofenac, paracetamol is relatively free of side effects and can be given to the elderly, those with kidney problems, allergies, gastric problems and other comorbidities.

Paracetamol can safely be given for longer durations as in long-lasting chronic pain associated with headaches, arthritis, back and cancer pain. The NSAIDs, as stated earlier, have analgesic and anti-inflammatory effects but need to be used with caution, especially in high-risk cases. Whatever be the analgesic, due consideration should be given to the age of the patient, body weight, presence of allergies, concurrent medications and presence of comorbidities such as diabetes, liver dysfunction, cardiac and neurological problems.

If pain does not respond to step 1 drugs, the next line of treatment are the weak opioids (tramadol and tapentadol), which are the step 2 drugs of the WHO analgesic ladder (Fig 7.1). These drugs are used to treat pain of moderate intensity. They act by binding on specific receptors called opioid receptors and block the passage of the pain impulse to the brain, although it is less potent than the strong opioids. They also act on the descending inhibitory pathway of pain by increasing good beneficial neurochemicals like serotonin and norepinephrine. Thus, they have a dual method of producing pain relief. These drugs are more easily accessible from pharmacies and chemists, as compared to morphine and other strong opioids, and are safe analgesics well-suited for treatment of moderate pain.

Opioids for chronic and intractable pain—boon or bane: Strong opioids are prescribed as step 3 of the WHO analgesic ladder and are used for treatment of severe pain. As mentioned earlier, the WHO by endorsing the analgesic ladder, has literally legitimized the use of strong opioids like morphine, fentanyl, buprenorphine and methadone for severe cancer pain. In this respect, it has been a boon for cancer patients. Even at the end of their lives, they can be free of pain and die with dignity. The other advantage of opioids like morphine is that they can be given orally and, therefore, are suitable for domiciliary pain management. Moreover, opioids like morphine and methadone are not expensive and, hence, easily affordable by the economically weaker sections of society.

Care needs to be taken while prescribing opioids. This includes screening of the patient for a history of substance use disorder and psychological/psychiatric disorders, especially when used for chronic non-cancer pain. And like all medications, the age of the person and presence of comorbidities should be kept in mind while prescribing it.

The use of opioids has some drawbacks. Firstly, patients tend to develop tolerance to the drug. This means that there is a progressive diminution of efficacy of the drug over a period of time and higher doses may be required to get the desired pain relief. Secondly, side effects such as sedation, involuntary movements and delirium preclude further escalation of dose with increasing pain. People complain of being *'horizontal and zoned out'* when they are on opioids although they admit that it kept the *'pain covered as with a thick blanket'*. Lastly, people develop physical dependence on opioids, which implies, that when these drugs are suddenly stopped they get withdrawal symptoms. This will not occur if the drug is slowly tapered off and then stopped.

An unfortunate adverse effect of opioids is developing psychological dependence that leads to addiction or craving for the drug despite the harm it is causing the person. In fact, opioid usage has been in the limelight for the wrong reasons as the 'opioid epidemic' in the US is claiming nearly 130 lives a day.[2] According to the US' Centers for Disease Control and Prevention (CDC), the death rate from opioid overdoses tripled from 6.1 per 100,000 people in 1999 to 19.8 in 2016.[3] Thus, large-scale use of opioid drugs has both personal and societal risks. Fortunately, in India, opioids are mainly used for treating cancer pain and, very rarely, for non-cancer pain and, hence, fatalities due to opioid use are not common.

We have discussed the medical management of chronic pain due to tissue injury (nociceptive pain). But neuropathic pain, which is pain due to disease or lesion in the nervous system, is an important cause of debilitating chronic pain that may only partially respond to the analgesics mentioned above. Neuropathic pain usually responds to 'non-analgesic' adjuvant medications such as anticonvulsants and antidepressants. It is called 'non-analgesic' because its primary use is for treatment of convulsions and depression respectively. But these drugs have analgesic properties that are beneficial for treatment of neuropathic pain. Anticonvulsant drugs include the gabapentinoids like gabapentin and pregabalin. Sedation, dizziness, fatigue and weight gain are some of the side effects of anticonvulsant drugs and caution needs to be exercised especially for elderly patients. Commonly used antidepressant drugs for treatment of chronic neuropathic pain are amitriptyline and nortriptyline. These drugs can cause sedation, dry mouth, vision abnormalities, constipation, urinary retention and cardiac abnormalities, and should be used with caution for certain patients. The other class of antidepressant drugs for neuropathic pain are those that block the receptors for serotonin and norepinephrine. Increasing their levels in the body activates the descending inhibitory pain pathway and, thus, relieves pain. These include duloxetine and venlafaxine among others.

Some medications for chronic pain can be applied on the skin as patches (transdermal) or some can be placed under the tongue (sublingual). Lignocaine (local anaesthetic) patches have been found to be effective for the incapacitating pain of post-herpetic neuralgia. Capsaicin, the active component of chilli pepper, has also been used in the form of skin patches, creams and gels for the treatment of neuropathic pain. Besides these, NSAIDs (like diclofenac and ketoprofen) and certain opioids (such as fentanyl and buprenorphine) are available as transdermal patches. Strong opioids like fentanyl are available as a lollipop that can be sucked for quick pain relief (oral transmucosal fentanyl citrate). Another strong opioid, buprenorphine, is available both as a skin patch and as a tablet that can be placed inside the mouth or under the tongue.

However, let me put in a word of caution for our dear readers. Please do not resort to self-medication and take these medicines *only* when prescribed by your doctor.

Interventional management of chronic pain

Sometimes it may be necessary to supplement medications with an interventional technique to provide relief to patients with chronic pain. These interventions are usually done by pain specialists and range from simple injections of local anaesthetic to more complicated neuromodulation techniques. Let us discuss the more commonly used interventional pain management modalities for chronic pain, which can broadly be classified as basic and advanced interventions.

Basic interventions for chronic pain management:

a. *Trigger point injections, dry needling and Botox injections*: Trigger point injections are injections of local anaesthetics given into the painful knots in the muscles or localized areas of tenderness. It may or may not be combined with steroids. It is used to treat a wide variety of patients with myofascial pain in the neck, shoulders, back and even for tender areas in widespread pain conditions as in fibromyalgia.

Dry needling is another modality that is useful for treating myofascial pain and muscle spasms. It is a technique that inserts fine needles of various lengths into the affected muscle to produce relaxation of the muscle and release spasm. The advantage of this method is that it does not require any kind of anaesthesia, can be performed in the outpatient department and lacks the side effects of medications. Pain specialists are increasingly using dry needling to treat back pain, sciatica, neck and shoulder and myofascial pain.

Similarly, Botox injection is also being widely used to treat myofascial pain, headaches, arthritis and neuropathic pain. In addition, it is also used to treat pain due to spasticity of muscles such as in neurological disorders like stroke, brain trauma, multiple sclerosis and cerebral palsy. Very often a combination of trigger point injections, dry needling and Botox injections are used to treat several chronic pain conditions.

b. *Nerve blocks*: Sometimes a nerve gets impinged or gets affected by disease and this can result in neuralgias or neuropathic pain. An example is a condition called meralgia paraesthetica, in which the nerve supplying the outer aspect of the thigh is entrapped in the groin, leading to burning pain, loss of sensation and tingling sensation in the outer aspect of the thigh. This usually occurs in people who wear tight belts or those with a pendulous abdomen. For such patients a targeted nerve block with steroids is given near the affected nerve to relieve the symptoms. These nerve blocks are administered using ultrasound to guide the trajectory of the injection for accuracy of the block as well as to prevent collateral injury to adjacent vital structures such as blood vessels and the nerve itself.

c. *Epidural steroid injections*: These are given either for chronic pain in the neck or low back, with or without radiation, to the arms or legs respectively. The various chronic pain conditions for which epidural injections are given include disc prolapse, pressure on the nerves exiting from the spinal cord to the upper and lower limbs due to degenerative changes in the cervical or lumbar spine, narrowing of the spinal canal (lumbar canal stenosis) and for persisting pain following spine surgery (failed back surgery syndrome).

The efficacy of epidural steroid injections, however, depends on proper patient selection, the underlying disease, duration of chronic pain (the longer the duration of symptoms, the less effective would be the injection), use of a contrast dye to facilitate accurate placement of the needle on the affected area and the right approach to the targeted area. It has been found that epidural injections in selected patients can obviate the need for hospitalization and spine surgery in the short-term.[4] Needless to say, an epidural injection is not a magic bullet and is only part of a multimodal treatment regime, which includes medications, dry needling, physical therapy and psychosocial therapies.

A case study would help illustrate this point.

Mrs Nandita was 50 years old and came in a wheelchair to the Pain Clinic during the Covid-19 pandemic. For two weeks, she had been having severe back pain radiating down her left leg, associated with difficulty in standing and walking. She was neither able to lie down flat on her back nor could she sleep because of the pain. She was anxious and fearful that this pain would cause her severe disability and cripple her forever. Clinical features revealed evidence of slipped disc (prolapsed intervertebral disc) in her lumbar spine and this was corroborated by MRI findings, which revealed the offending disc in the lower lumbar spine compressing the nerve to her left leg.

She had consulted a spine surgeon who advised her spine surgery, but she was dead against it because she feared that it would make her permanently bedridden. Besides her anxiety related to severe pain, the then Covid-19 pandemic was further increasing her anxiety. Even while interacting with us, she repeatedly kept sanitizing her hands. After reassuring her and assuaging her anxiety, she was started on treatment using the multimodality approach, comprising medications, dry needling, epidural steroid injection near the affected nerve root (transforaminal injection), physiotherapy and psychotherapy.

Besides the above mentioned therapies, some back exercises were taught to her, which she was encouraged to do as part of her daily routine at home. She responded well to this line of management and not only got relief from pain but also gradually started to walk without any support, was able to do her household chores and slowly resumed her normal life.

One of the drawbacks of epidural steroid injections is the limited duration of action of steroid and consequently the temporariness of pain relief. But it must be kept in mind that the relief of pain obtained by steroid injection should be utilized for initiating a complete rehabilitation programme comprising exercises, physiotherapy modalities and suitable physical activities that would enable the body's own healing process to kick in and provide longer-lasting pain relief.

The other steroid injection commonly given for chronic pain is into joints. Joint injections include injections into the knee joint for osteoarthritis in the knees, shoulder joint for frozen shoulder, facet joints for low back pain (facets connect one vertebra to the other) and sacroiliac joint (which connects the spine with the pelvis) for back pain. These again provide only temporary respite from pain, and should be supplemented by exercises and physiotherapy for longer-lasting relief.

Advanced interventions for chronic pain management:

a. *Radiofrequency [RF] ablation*: is done to address the neural (nerve) component of chronic pain. In this procedure, a high frequency electric current from a generator passes through an insulated needle producing heat at its tip. When the tip of the needle is placed near the affected nerve, it creates a small lesion in the nerve, burning the nerve and, thus, interrupts the pain signals emanating from it.

Depending on the heat generated, there are various types of radiofrequency (RF) ablation. **Conventional RF** uses heat in the range of 80°C, which destroys the nerves by burning them and, thus, produces pain relief. In **Cooled RF**, a cooling system is incorporated around the probe so that greater amount of RF energy can be delivered at lower temperatures. In **Pulsed RF**, the energy is delivered in pulses so that the temperature is dissipated and not allowed to increase beyond 42°C and, as a result, the nerve is not ablated but is, rather, 'shocked'. This is a more patient-friendly technique, as it does not damage the nerves like conventional RF and can at the same time provide pain relief for three to six months.

Radiofrequency ablation is commonly used to treat a wide variety of chronic pain conditions, including back pain due to degenerative spine disease, osteoarthritis knee, facial pains due to neuralgias, etc.

b. *Neuromodulation*: When chronic neuropathic pain is unresponsive to medications and basic interventional procedures, advanced procedures like neuromodulation therapies can be considered. Neuromodulation employs highly sophisticated medical technologies to alter nerve activity by targeted delivery of either an electrical stimulus or a chemical agent (drug) at specific sites on or near the spinal cord to modulate pain. There is a whole range of neuromodulation therapies available for chronic pain management, but the three most commonly used are: electrical stimulation of the spinal cord (spinal cord stimulation); dorsal root ganglion (DRG) stimulation; and intrathecal pumps for intraspinal delivery of opioids.

In **spinal cord stimulation**, electrodes are placed on the surface of the spinal cord between its outer covering and the vertebral column in the epidural space. These electrodes are connected by wires to a generator that is implanted under the skin, much like a pacemaker. These deliver low-voltage electrical impulses through the electrodes to the target site on the spinal cord corresponding to the area of pain. The sensation so generated masks the actual pain felt by the patient and, thus, modulates the pain. Spinal cord stimulation is used in patients with intractable neuropathic pain due to failed back surgery syndrome, chronic regional pain syndrome, peripheral neuropathies and phantom limb pain. Before the final implantation of the stimulator a trial period of stimulation is done, and only if that is effective, is the final implantation performed.

Dorsal root ganglion stimulation is used for patients with intractable neuropathic pain of the upper or lower extremities. The electrodes are placed near the dorsal root ganglion of the affected nerve, close to the spinal cord (see figure 2.2), so that focused stimulation can be done for a specific area of pain.

Intrathecal pumps or **intraspinal drug delivery systems** are programmable devices that deliver small doses of opioids as a continuous infusion into the intrathecal space, which contains the cerebrospinal fluid that bathes the spinal cord. This is done from a pump or reservoir that contains the medicine and is implanted under the skin, much like a pacemaker, and which contains the medication. The pump is connected to the cerebrospinal fluid space by a catheter. It is usually given to terminal cancer patients with intractable pain, who have responded well to oral opioids but who need increasing doses and have unacceptable side effects with high doses of opioids. By delivering a very small dose (1/300) of the oral dose directly to the target organ (opioid receptors in the spinal cord), the side effects of high doses of opioids can be considerably reduced. But, just as with spinal cord stimulation, before implanting the device, a trial of the drug is given and only if this produces a satisfactory response is the actual pump implanted. It is also necessary to rule out any substance use disorder before undertaking to do the procedure.

The main disadvantages of neuromodulation devices are the prohibitively high cost and the technical expertise required to perform the procedure and maintain the devices.

Treating the Body

Healthcare professionals, most often, tend to focus on the biomedical aspects for treating pain, using drugs and pain interventions and not focus on non-pharmacological strategies such as physical activity, physical therapy, adequate sleep, nutrition and even occupational health. Let us discuss some of these non-pharmacological methods of treatment for chronic pain that are frequently used for treating the body.

Physical Activity and Physical Therapy

Since the 1980s, physicians treating pain have advocated moving away from the policy of 'rest' to minimizing rest and remaining active. Besides being beneficial for pain, physical activity improves the physical and mental health of the individual, including depression, physical deconditioning and obesity. The various components of proper neuromuscular function include strength, muscular and aerobic endurance, power, agility, balance and flexibility. Man operates under the *'law of use: use it or lose it.'* Since both bone and soft tissues remodel depending on the stress imposed on them, exercise is important not only for treatment but also for prevention of chronic pain. Thus, physical therapy and activity are key components of a chronic pain rehabilitation programme.

The physiotherapist plays an important role in the multidisciplinary management and restoration of physical function in a patient with chronic pain. Besides doing physical therapy, the role of the physiotherapist is also to educate the patient about their pain and the benefits of the therapy being given. A recent study found that pain neurophysiology education, when combined with therapeutic exercises to treat chronic low back pain, was more effective than therapeutic exercises used alone.[5] We did the same for Mrs Nandita (case mentioned earlier) and impressed upon her to continue with the exercise even after the sessions with the physiotherapist were over, to ensure long-lasting relief. More often than not, doctors and physiotherapists enumerate a list of exercises that need to be done and even demonstrate them, but how often do they educate their patients on the benefits of exercise and the rationale behind the exercises?

Physiotherapists advise and prescribe exercises that include strengthening, stretching and core exercises depending on their physical assessment of the patient. These are usually started in a graded way so that the patient can tolerate them and not end up with more pain. In fact, the National Institute for Health and Care Excellence's (NICE) osteoarthritis guidelines state that, '...exercise should be a core treatment ... irrespective of age, comorbidity, pain severity and disability. Exercise should include: local muscle strengthening and general aerobic fitness.'[6]

Manual therapy and myofascial release are some of the modalities that physiotherapists use to mobilize stiff joints and release muscles and nerves. Besides these, the other modalities include heat and cold therapy, electrical stimulation, laser and ultrasound. Kinesiophobia and fear-avoidance are major factors that physiotherapists have to contend with while managing patients with chronic pain, and counselling and patience are key in handling these.

Sleep disorders

Sleep disorders can be a cause or consequence of chronic pain and, therefore, need to be managed. This can be done with both pharmacological and non-pharmacological methods. Many a time, patients suffering from chronic pain may require medications like sedatives, antidepressants or anti-anxiety drugs so that they can have undisturbed sleep. Pharmacologically, the drugs of choice for insomnia are melatonin and the antidepressants. The latter are particularly useful, as they have additional analgesic properties as well.

Among the non-pharmacological strategies, cognitive behaviour therapy (CBT) has been found to be useful. It is a structured programme that helps in identifying the thoughts and behaviours that aggravate sleep disorders. These thoughts are modified to promote better sleep patterns. Other methods that are combined with CBT to promote sleep, include sleep hygiene, stimulus control, sleep restriction, improved environmental surroundings, relaxation training and passive awakening.

Knowledge and practice of sleep hygiene methods in particular is a useful non-pharmacological strategy in patients with chronic pain. The following steps of sleep hygiene have been found to be useful.

a. Arise at the same time each morning.
b. Limit daily 'in-bed' time.
c. Limit or discontinue stimulants of the central nervous system like caffeine, alcohol and nicotine before bedtime.
d. Avoid daytime napping.
e. Exercise every day, but not just prior to sleep time.
f. Avoid emotionally charged stimulation near bedtime. Read or listen to radio, instead of using other electronic devices.
g. Keep to regular meal timings and avoid a large meal just before bedtime.
h. Relaxation techniques to induce sleep can be practiced.
i. Sleeping conditions should be comfortable.

Last but not the least, if pain is the cause of sleeplessness, it is advisable to take an analgesic.

Nutrition

'Let food be thy medicine…'—Hippocrates

The connection between nutrition and chronic pain has often been ignored in the past. But this ancient saying by Hippocrates has proven to be true and, today, the focus has shifted back on the role of nutrition in prevention of chronic pain. In fact, nutrition is now a part of the multidisciplinary management of pain. As mentioned earlier, many patients with chronic pain have a high level of pro-inflammatory cytokines and, therefore, consuming food and nutrients that have anti-inflammatory properties could be beneficial. A diet low in fibre and micro-nutrients tends to be pro-inflammatory, whereas a diet rich in fibre, healthy oils, fruits, vegetables, whole grains and low in sugar is anti-inflammatory.

Similarly, omega-3 fats have been shown to be beneficial in patients with rheumatoid arthritis with lesser need for anti-inflammatory drugs and should be included in the diet for these patients.[7] Tubers, turmeric and ginger also have anti-inflammatory properties. Turmeric, which contains curcumin, is a yellow extract from the root of a plant largely found in Asia and Central America. It has antioxidant and analgesic properties that are useful in inflammatory and joint diseases besides being a digestive aid. Alongside nutrients, adequate water intake is also important for patients with chronic pain.

All of this leads to the question as to whether there is an optimal diet for patients with chronic pain. Given the pro-inflammatory properties of certain foods—and the anti-inflammatory effects of certain others—researchers have made a hypothetical nutritional pyramid to serve as an integrative tool for patients with chronic pain.[8] The base of the pyramid is water intake of 1.5 to 2 litres, and ascending upwards in order of priority are fruits and vegetables, whole grains, extra virgin olive oil, red wine and yoghurt. On top of the pyramid are foods that need to be avoided, which includes poultry, red or processed meat and sweets. Besides this, daily nutritional supplementation of vitamin D3, B12 and omega-3 fats need to be taken as well.

Nutraceuticals are getting popular for a variety of conditions ranging from cardiac disease to neurodegenerative conditions like Alzheimer's disease. Nutraceuticals are a combination of nutritional and pharmaceutical products taken as dietary supplements that provide medical or health benefits in the prevention and treatment of various conditions. Some nutraceuticals used for chronic pain include vitamin D, calcium supplements and glucosamine combined with chondroitin sulphate. The latter is useful for osteoarthritis of the knees. Acetyl-L-carnitine (ALC) and acetyl lipoic acid (ALA) have been used for chronic pain due to neuropathies, like diabetic neuropathy- and chemotherapy-induced neuropathy.

Treating the Mind

Psychological Therapies

Since most patients with chronic pain and chronic pain syndrome have many psychological issues, treating the mind is an important aspect of the multidisciplinary management of pain. After the psychological assessment of the patient, a fairly clear picture emerges as to which behaviours and thoughts need to be targeted. Accordingly, those psychotherapies are selected that would be most effective in least number of sessions.

In principle, the rule of seeing the patient is once in a week, and with betterment, the sessions are staggered to once in fifteen days. With further improvement, the frequency of sessions is slowly reduced and eventually faded out and stopped. Subsequently, patients are called for regular follow-ups to, essentially, reinforce the 'healthy' learned behaviours and ease out any new difficulties.

Psychological interventions may be required in case of any emergencies like suicidal ideation or any crisis situations. However, crisis management using psychological interventions is not encouraged with chronic pain patients as they tend to develop dependency on the clinical psychologist instead of being in the driver's seat themselves.

Broadly, psychotherapies that are effective with patients with chronic pain and chronic pain syndrome can be categorized as behaviour therapies, cognitive therapies, stress inoculation, acceptance and commitment therapy, problem-solving strategies and supportive psychotherapies.

Behaviour therapies

Behaviour therapies are based on learning principles. The basic premise is that behaviours are learned, hence, they can be unlearned and new behaviours learned. Thus, those behaviours deemed unhealthy can be changed by replacing them with new behaviours that are adaptive and beneficial to the patient. The focus of the behaviour therapies is on the 'here and now' situations rather than delving deep into the psyche of the person. These therapies are effective with any age group and with varying intellectual functioning, even with patients with cognitive decline.

Behaviour therapy to promote relaxation: Most chronic pain patients report having tensed muscles, either due to pain or stress or a combination of the two. Relaxation therapies are helpful not only in easing the tensed muscles but help when pain is associated with insomnia, anxiety, post-traumatic stress disorder and hypertension. There are a variety of techniques, but only those will be described here that have been found to be most effective.

   a. *Jacobson's Progressive Muscular Relaxation (JPMR)*:[9] This technique uses, alternatively, the method of tensing and relaxing small groups of muscles in a systematic manner. A group of muscles are tightened followed by the relaxation phase, with the release of the tensed muscles. Usually, one starts from the extremities and then covers the whole body. It takes about 15–20 minutes to complete it, by the end of which the body and mind feel relaxed. Preferably, JPMR should be done very slowly in a semi-darkened room and noise-free environment.
   b. *Visualization or imagery*:[10] involves use of imagination to relax the body and mind. As negative thoughts regarding our pain disturb our mental state by making us angry or anxious,

so do pleasant and calming thoughts bring back peace and relaxation. Using this premise, the visualization method uses mental images to promote calmness within a person. In this relaxation technique, the person is encouraged to form a visual journey to a peaceful place or situation. As far as possible many senses like touch, smell, sound and sight are incorporated for vivid and vibrant images to be formed. When a person visualizes calming images on a regular basis, it increases the focusing ability of the mind and, when distressed with pain, is able to transport self mentally to a pleasing situation.

c. *Autogenic training*:[11] is another relaxation method. It teaches the body to follow one's own verbal command. These commands 'instruct' the body to relax. The verbal cues induce sensations of heaviness, warmth and coolness. The six established techniques are inducing heaviness in the body, inducing warmth, heart practice to focus on heartbeat, breathing practice to focus on breathing and abdominal practice to pay attention to abdominal sensations. Imagery is used and the person is asked to imagine self in a peaceful environment like a garden or in the mountains. This method is useful for achieving deep relaxation in conditions like panic attacks, hypervigilance, sleep deprivation and hypertension. This brings peace to a troubled mind.

d. *Biofeedback*:[12] is used in conjunction with other relaxation techniques. It is done with the help of machines that give the patient feedback related to bodily functions like temperature, heart rate, breathing, muscle contraction, sweat gland activity and even brain waves. The feedback helps the person to control and change these parameters so that they are able to relax themselves. It is effective with migraine headaches, chronic pains like fibromyalgia, spasm in certain muscle groups, high blood pressure, chemotherapy side effects, stroke, anxiety and stress.

e. *Meditation*: Among the complementary and alternative methods that induce relaxation, meditation is a useful method to become aware of bodily sensations and mental activities without being judgemental about them. Most meditation techniques largely focus on breathing and repeating words or sounds. Amongst various types of meditation, mindfulness meditation is considered to be most effective in relaxing a person.[13] It is an efficacious relaxation technique for relieving pain. It trains the mind to calm itself by slowing down the pace of thoughts and letting go of negativity. The person is taught to observe self, particularly the pain, without attaching any meaning to it. This detachment of the emotional component from the pain experience quite often relieves the pain. The method uses techniques like deep breathing and creating awareness of the body and mind. Thus, one learns to accept one's feelings, thoughts and sensations in the 'now' situation without attaching undue meaning to it, or in other words, being non-judgemental about it. Apart from diminishing the pain experience, mindfulness meditation helps in reducing depressive feelings, too, by detaching the emotional surcharge related to chronic pain.

f. *Yoga*:[14] Also among the complementary and alternative methods, is this ancient Indian method of connecting mind and body. Yoga amalgamates stretching, breathing exercises and meditation. There are innumerable yoga postures for addressing pain in different parts of the body. Yoga therapy improves mobility and flexibility, prevents joint and cartilage deterioration, increases strength and stability in postures, promotes relaxation of both body and mind, reduces stress and, overall, seeks to provide holistic treatment of both physical and psychological ailments. It is especially useful in chronic conditions like fibromyalgia, back pain, neck pain, arthritis, migraine headaches and chronic fatigue syndrome. Since it elevates mood, it is useful in reducing stress, anxiety and depression.

Behaviour therapy to reduce anxiety

a. *Systematic Desensitization (SD):*[15] is a three-step method, namely learning a relaxation technique, building the anxiety hierarchy and connecting the stimulus to the incompatible response or counter conditioning. Let me illustrate how this method is used, citing Mrs Annu's case (chapter 3). In step one, she was trained to relax using JPMR. In step two, an anxiety hierarchy was built starting from the least anxiety-provoking situation to the maximum one. Then the anxiety ladder was worked upon, starting with a neutral situation and graduating to the least anxiety-provoking one. In step three, after every item on the ladder, Mrs Annu had to voluntarily bring down her anxiety by relaxing her tensed muscles. The tensed muscles were the response to the anxiety, whereas relaxation was the incompatible response or counter conditioning to the tensed muscles. In this way, the next higher level of anxiety-generating item in the hierarchy was worked upon, and the process was continued till the entire hierarchical list was complete. While working on the list, it reduced her hypervigilance and the almost phobic response to a fall.

Cognitive therapies for anxiety, depression and stress due to chronic pain

Cognitive Behaviour Therapy (CBT):[16] Amongst cognitive therapies, CBT has empirically been found to be efficacious for pain management. It aims to change the way a person views pain (pain perception), alter the thoughts, emotions and behaviours related to pain and build up better coping strategies than the ones being used earlier. CBT directs the person's awareness to the fact that the control lies with him/her. This is done by challenging the automatic beliefs and implementing practical means to change and modify beliefs and behaviour. It is most effective in reducing cognitions related to depression, anxiety, chronic pain and stress.

Before one starts with CBT sessions, it is important to find the distorted thoughts and pain-related cognitions. Some of these are the following:

a. *Catastrophizing*: Thoughts assuming the 'worst is happening' are found in a substantial number of pain patients. These thoughts could be like 'no one can help me, my pain will forever be like this', 'there is no help for pain', 'my pain will go only once I die', 'these twinges in my leg and back tell me that other parts of my body are getting affected' and so on.

b. *Polarized thinking*: is when thoughts are based on dichotomous choices as 'good' and 'bad' or 'black' and 'white', without any 'shades of grey' being an option. For example, 'I will never be able to walk or run as I used to, so why make an attempt' or 'there is no point in working because I cannot work as I used to before'.

c. *Filtering*: is when negative thoughts get magnified and positive thoughts are filtered out, thereby minimizing positivity. For instance, despite completing the purchases at a grocery store, the person still says, 'My pain was so bad while shopping for groceries that I can never go shopping.' Thus, filtering out the recovery and not acknowledging her improved functionality in completing shopping.

d. *Personalization*: is the tendency to relate everything to self. The distortion lies in the interpretation of each experience, conversation, remark or even a look as an indication of one's self-worth. One takes the responsibility for events where none is required. For instance, 'My pain drove my wife away as, naturally, who would want to live with a man crippled with pain.'
e. *Overgeneralization*: is when a conclusion is drawn based on a single incident or piece of evidence. The person tries to avoid future disappointments by inhibiting any activity based on conclusions drawn from a previous incident. This leads to a restricted life. For instance, 'Everyone was laughing and joking instead of asking about my welfare, and so I would rather not meet these people again.'
f. *Negative labelling*: is when one addresses oneself with negative words like 'failure', 'crippled', 'disabled' and so on.
g. *Emotional reasoning*: is when one believes something is true because one strongly believes in it. For example, in the first chapter Rahul had said, 'I'm destiny's child.'

In CBT, the above Automatic Negative Thoughts (ANTs)[17] are targeted where the words 'should' and 'must' are overused, thereby overriding other rational thoughts. These thoughts are challenged and attempted to be replaced with more realistic and positive ones. Let me illustrate by giving an excerpt from a therapeutic session with Mrs Annu (chapter 3).

Mrs Annu had unexpressed anger, as reflected on the psychological tests. Therefore, the first few therapeutic sessions were devoted to her expressing her own anguish by using the ventilation technique. During the second session, she expressed thoughts like 'no one cares for me'; 'my son loves his wife more than me'; 'I had sacrificed so much for my children, including giving up a career, but, in return, I get mistreated by my son', and more statements in the same vein.

Therapist (T): *Let us evaluate the statement 'no one loves me'. Would you like to elaborate it further?*

Mrs A: *Well, you see, ever since he got married, my son pays more attention to his wife and daughter.*

T: *That is only one person. You said that 'no one loves me'.*

Mrs A: *Is this not sufficient?*

T: *(Silent)*

Mrs A: *Okay, my younger son and my husband do care for me.*

T: *(nodding) Could you elaborate your daily activities with the family from morning onwards?*

Mrs A: *My husband, both sons and I have tea together on the front lawn. My sons joke around and try to make me laugh. It is a pleasant time for me because my daughter-in-law is not present. She is busy in readying her daughter for school. My elder son then goes to drop the child. Then all three men leave together for the factory and come back at the same time in the evening. We all have tea and snacks together. My elder son then joins his wife and daughter and they spend time together. We all have dinner, after that everyone is involved in their separate activities. My husband and I like watching some TV serials and so we retire to our room.*

T: *The entire family spends time together and the tradition of having family meals continues. Where do you feel the lack of attention or neglect?*

Mrs A: *Why does my son give more importance to his wife?*

T: *Please describe what does giving 'more attention' means to you.*

Mrs A: *(with a rather defiant look on her face was quiet)*

T: *(waited)*

Mrs A: Are you on their side?

T: (smilingly) I'm on nobody's side.

Mrs A: Okay, he gives me importance but I'm no longer first for him.

T: Let us understand this statement of being first.

Mrs A: (thoughtfully) He does spend time with me. Are you suggesting that I'm jealous?

T: (Smilingly) Would you also like to evaluate your love for your son?

Mrs A: I love my son unconditionally.

T: Naturally. So as a mother what do you wish for your son?

Mrs A: Being happy.

T: What do you think will make him happy?

Mrs A: A successful career and a successful marriage.

T: Do you think this is happening?

Mrs A: No, my anger is spoiling his life. I'm being a bad mother.

T: Let us not use labels. Would you like to summarize your understanding of your feelings at this juncture?

Mrs A: You have made me acknowledge that I have been angry because my son made his own choice while marrying. My family cares for me and gives me time.

T: (silent)

Mrs A: (thoughtfully) I have realized that my anger with my son got displaced on my daughter-in-law and granddaughter. Instead of being angry with him, I remain angry with her. This has made me distressed and unhappy. In turn, I believe I have made others unhappy. My anger and tensions are making me unwell. I think I realize the link between my anger and my pains.

T: How does this revelation help you?

Mrs A: I think I need to work upon my anger.

Some anger controlling techniques were then discussed. Homework was given to practice these techniques and keep a check on her 'anger-related thoughts'.

Similarly, her feelings and communication with her daughter-in-law were handled. She understood how her emotions were affecting her physically and psychologically, thereby increasing her pains.

As discussed above, CBT is an effective technique with depression too. In fact, it is the therapy of choice with depressive cognitions and ruminations. It was used successfully with Mrs Soma (chapter 3). This along with medical and physical therapies improved her mood as well as her pain. As a result, she became more functional and slowly resumed some of her duties.

Stress Inoculation Therapy (SIT):[18] This involves exposing the patient to increasing levels of perceived stress, so that an effort is made to use different coping skills to keep stress under control. This gradually helps in building tolerance or immunity to that particular stressor. Several methods are used, namely deep muscle relaxation, cognitive restructuring, breathing exercises, assertiveness skills, thought-stopping, role-playing and guided self-dialogue. The SIT is helpful in managing stress, post-traumatic stress disorder, anxiety and chronic conditions like pain.

Acceptance and Commitment Therapy (ACT):[19,20] Here the therapist does not aim to decrease chronic pain, instead the focus is on helping a person to change their behaviour. It uses mindfulness-based intervention and blends it with commitment, behavioural and cognitive change strategies. The six tenets it uses are willingness to accept, cognitive defusion, contact with the present moment, observing the self, values and committed action. The person is encouraged to reorganize their efforts and reduce the focus from eliminating pain, to becoming actively involved in meaningful activities that one cares for and cherishes in life.

While using ACT with chronic pain patients, the therapist helps the patient to: (a) accept experiences instead of rejecting them because of fear of developing pain; (b) choose behaviours mindfully, instead of reacting in a set pattern (automatic) or having a conditioned response; and (c) taking actions in consonance with the valued goals, instead of being stymied with pain-related thoughts and its accompanying emotions and feelings. The aim is to increase psychological flexibility.

a. *Acceptance*: of pain does not mean giving up hope or surrender to pain, rather it means increasing psychological flexibility. This is to promote openness to experiences in order to continue bringing changes to behaviours as and when the opportunities arise, which are in accordance to one's valued ideas. To increase the acceptance of their condition, one needs to be non-judgemental, acknowledge the pain, focus on self and learn to find the good in the situation. Hence, therapists build willingness skills, which help the patient accept that the distressing emotions and negative thoughts are natural to pain, but at the same time, life cannot be put on hold for fear of pain and imagined safety. *Writing experiences where similar thoughts and emotions were felt, and how the patient had overcome it in return for something that was cherished—is a simple exercise. Doing this exercise takes away the significance attached to pain, that was being harboured by the patient.*

b. *Defusion*: is the next step, in which the person is encouraged to only observe their thoughts without attaching any meaning or significance to it. This helps in distancing or dissociating oneself from the emotional implications attached to those thoughts. A frequently used exercise is labelling the thought. For example, if the thought is *'I have tremendous pain in my back'*, one prefixes this thought with a phrase like *'I think I have tremendous pain in my back'* or it can be made longer as *'Today I'm getting the thought that I think I have tremendous pain in my back'*. The patient is then asked how he/she is feeling and whether the thought feels a part of him/her. When this process is repeated innumerable times, the emotion laden sentences lose their power to hurt.

c. *Present moment awareness*: is enhanced by concentrating on the moment instead of ruminating about past experiences or future fears. This is accomplished by mindfulness accompanied by use of all senses. With deep breathing the person's attention is diverted to *seeing* a flower or picture in the room or *hearing* the song of the birds or *smelling* the flowers or *touching* the softness of the carpet or rug.

d. *Self as context*: is the ability to view oneself objectively as if one is observing oneself. Self is considered as separate from one's thoughts, emotions, feelings and physical body. The premise for this separation is that self or identity tends to get interlinked with pain. As we saw in Mrs Ankita's case described above, over a period of time, pain became her 'alter ego'. Hence, while viewing self as separate from pain, the person learns to observe pain without becoming their own pain.

e. *Values*: represent the goals that the person wants to work towards despite the pain.

f. *Committed actions*: are determined efforts to change the behaviour.

These strivings increase psychological flexibility as one becomes more adaptable to situations, able to reorganize thoughts, shift mental paradigms and able to maintain equilibrium between conflicting emotions, desires and various domains of life.

ACT was used for Mrs Ankita's chronic pain due to fibromyalgia, along with medications and physical therapy. She responded well to the therapy and now engages in several cherished goals. She has recently completed a distance learning course on counselling psychology and is learning to play the guitar. She is actively involved in the upbringing of her seven-year-old daughter, which she was unable to do earlier. She has also gone back to her singing practice in the morning. Today, despite her pain, she is leading a more committed and happier life, instead of lying in bed with hot packs and pain being her constant companion.

Supportive psychotherapies: Supportive psychotherapeutic methods[21,22] help to stabilize day-to-day functions, bring emotional equilibrium, strengthen adaptability by building up the coping mechanism and are useful in reducing the distress of the patient without delving into the psychological and behavioural causes. Usually, they are an adjunct to other psychotherapeutic methods.

Some supportive methods are: guidance, tension control and release, environmental manipulation, externalization of interests, reassurance, prestige suggestion, pressure and coercion, persuasion and ventilation. Patients with pain are particularly benefited by ventilation, tension control and release, reassurance, environmental manipulation, persuasion and externalization of interests. Let us discuss them in more detail.

    a. *Ventilation*: is one of the first methods to be used for the patient to be able to vent out powerful emotions. When it is done in the presence of an uncritical and non-judgemental person, these pent-up emotions, fears, conflicts, worries, anxieties, unfulfilled hopes and ambitions lose their frightening quality. The repeated disclosures desensitize or lessen the emotional tinge from situations, thus robbing the negativity related to them. An emotional catharsis then takes place, releasing the person from certain held beliefs that had been detrimental to their well-being. In the case of Mrs Annu (chapter 3), we devoted two sessions to using the ventilation technique to help her pour out her feelings of anger, disappointment and frustrations before other methods like CBT were used.

b. *Tension control and release*: Tension belongs to the anxiety spectrum but is of lesser intensity and is not pathological like anxiety seen in anxiety disorders. However, pervasive tensions are detrimental to the well-being of a person and, hence, need to be reduced. Tensions can be relieved by relaxation techniques, meditation, self-hypnosis, massage and electrical stimulation.

c. *Reassurance*: It works wonders with anxious and depressed persons. When the person has doubts about not getting better or pain leading to disability, reassurance gives solace to the sufferer. When fears are openly discussed and explanations are offered, it often belies the distorted thoughts that the patient carries. Reassurance, thus, helps to divert the patient's mind from self-destructive thoughts, eases their anxiety and guides them towards self-improving mechanisms.

d. *Environmental manipulation*: As many chronic pain patients do have relationship issues, conflicts and hostilities, it helps if changes are made in the environment around the patient. Many patients feel that they have no right to openly make demands, or they think that their life situation is unalterable and cannot be changed. In such cases, a change in the environment by moving the person to a more congenial and less threatening situation is preferable. A change in scene, meeting new people, socializing and being involved in other activities distracts the person in a positive way.

e. *Persuasion*: It is a powerful technique for the person to whom reasoning and logic is appealing. The attempt is to persuade and motivate the person to recognize that they have a power within themselves to get better. Hence, an appeal is made to the person's intelligence and reasoning ability.

f. *Externalization of interests*: Distress, anxiety, depression and a preoccupation with pain symptoms foster withdrawal from pursuit of interests and diversions that are part of healthy normal living. Indulgence in various activities takes away the constant worry and fixation over the pain experience. Thus, the patient is encouraged to engage in hobbies, recreational activities and creative arts. These include art, music, dance, drama therapy and journalling. We can see how in Mrs Ankita's case singing and learning to play a musical instrument helped in easing her pain.

- *Art Therapy*: Art is one of the most powerful ways of emotional catharsis where pent up emotions are expressed through creative activity. As the adage goes, 'a picture is worth a thousand words', so is the worth of this therapy to help release emotions not otherwise expressed. Depending upon the inclination of the person, colours, pencils, charcoal or crayons are used.
- *Music Therapy*: Music has a soothing effect on the mind. It provides sensory stimulation that induces a response, which relaxes the body and mind, increases rhythmic breathing and induces rest and mental relief.
- *Dance/Movement Therapy (DMT)*: is a mind/body integrative form of psychotherapy that combines dance,

movement, emotional expression and creativity. The rhythmic and guided movements reduce pain as it improves posture, gait, mobility and release of tension in a more amusing and entertaining manner. It improves both physical and emotional well-being as it leads to more socializing, serves to distract, increases confidence and concentration and helps in emotional regulation.

Chronic pain patients who have strong fear-avoidance behaviour, learn to move their body through guided therapy in a safe and relaxed setting under the supervision of a therapist. Most patients improve significantly with respect to resilience, body awareness, pain intensity and kinesiophobia (fear of movement), thereby reducing their stress levels too. Dance/Movement Therapy is also widely used with cancer patients, fibromyalgia and also the physically fatigued caregivers of cancer patients.

- *Drama Therapy*: This form of group therapy encourages the patient to emote through dramatic expressions and body movements while enacting real life situations and simultaneously overcoming the conflicts related to their roles. Chronic pain patients, while role-playing, are encouraged to emote and also to analyse self-behaviour, reflect on past and present situations, their relationships, any conflicts within themselves or with others and evaluate their stressors. Drama helps to release pent-up emotions and reduces frustration, anger, anxiety, depression, hostility and stress. Moreover, when role reversal is enacted, the patient is able to visualize and understand the stress of family members. In this way, both the emotional and physical aspects of chronic pain are addressed.
- *Pain Diary*: This is a written record kept by the patient to track the frequency, intensity, duration, triggers,

management and time taken for reduction of pain. This is akin to headache diary, which is advocated for patients with migraine.

- *Emotional Diary*: Simultaneously, the patient is encouraged to maintain an 'Emotional Diary' where they record their emotional experiences while in pain, thoughts associated with pain and any event preceding the exacerbation of pain. While the Pain Diary is a useful record for the pain specialist to monitor the response to treatment, the Emotional Diary acts as a stress buster for the patient and gives clues to the clinical psychologist to target thoughts and emotions in psychotherapeutic sessions. After recording the stressful/negative experience, the patient is encouraged to write or remember a happy experience. The basic premise is to help the patient emote the negative emotions and allow catharsis to take place, while the happy experience keeps the mood positive.

In the next chapter, you will see how music, art and dance therapy were integrated in Rahul's pain rehabilitation programme.

Social therapies

Family therapy: is essential in most cases, especially if there are expressed emotions (hostility) towards the sufferer. Most families have added burden of extra work and responsibilities as well as dealing with emotional fluctuations of the patient. Families could also face curtailment of ambitions and opportunities, forfeiting their own careers and diminishing hopes of life returning to normalcy. In such a scenario, family therapy is strongly indicated. Three types of family therapies[23,24] are useful, namely structural, operant-behavioural and cognitive behavioural.

a. *Structural Family Therapy*: focuses on pain in a family member acting as a balance in a dysfunctional family. Such family systems resist change and seek balance within the family by rigidly adhering to family rules. These families are known as 'psychosomatic families' with some characteristics like: enmeshment with weak ego boundaries; being overprotective, with oversolicitous behaviour towards the patient; rigidity and inflexibility in ascribed roles; and lack of insight into the dysfunctionality within the family. Insight is necessary for any resolution to take place.[25] In such families, pain serves the purpose of maintaining family homeostasis by encouraging 'sick role homeostasis', which means the role of patient and caregiver get assigned for creating some semblance of balance in the family. Pain also upholds psuedo-mutuality or superficial appearance of openness in the family though the relationships are rigid and communication skewed. Therapy is directed towards breaking these mindsets, dealing with the actual dysfunctionality rather than cloaking it and having direct communication. The emphasis is on achieving a sense of individuality so that growth in relationship happens.

b. *Operant Behavioural Therapy*:[26] is based on learning principles. Here the pain cues provided by the family, manifesting as oversolicitous behaviour, are recognized and curtailed. These may include over-responsiveness to expressions of pain, restricting accountability, taking over activities that the patient can do and passively acquiescing to avoidance behaviour. The family is advised not to shoulder unwanted responsibilities or undesirable activities that the patient does not want to do. The therapy targets these behaviours to be unlearned, and new and more adaptive behaviours to be learned. Care is taken during therapeutic sessions that hostility towards the patient is not generated.

c. *Cognitive Behavioural Transactional Process Therapy*:[27] first appraises the set belief system of the family regarding the pain, disability, stress and coping mechanism of the family. When the appraisals are positive and the family has many coping resources, the outcome is optimistic, whereas the reverse is seen when coping options are few and appraisals are threatening. The therapy, thus, focuses on challenging the belief system of the family, underscoring the importance of appraisals and its effect on the outcomes.

Marital therapy: is essential for most patients with chronic pain. Misunderstandings occur due to many reasons and they become a source of stress for both the patient and the spouse. Marital disharmony often leads to tensions in the entire family.

a. *Integrative Behavioural Couple Therapy*[28,29] *(IBCT)*: focuses on increasing the emotional acceptance and tolerance in the couple that includes empathic joining. This allows the patient to express their pain without levelling accusations at each other.

b. *Unified detachment*: This is another strategy, which helps the partners to distance themselves from emotion-laden discussions and try to intellectually analyse the problem. This robs the emotional surcharge associated with many situations at home and amongst themselves.

c. *Tolerance strategies*: employ finding the positive aspects even in negative situations as well as self-care behaviour during the session and in between sessions. This helps in distinguishing the adaptive behaviour from maladaptive ones.

Rahul and his wife responded well to IBCT with unified detachment strategy to cope with the acceptance of residual chronic pain with which Rahul and his wife would have had to live.

Group therapy: Group therapies primarily act as support groups for chronic pain patients. They traditionally use relaxation therapies, supportive psychotherapy methods and help develop problem-solving techniques. These groups not only act as emotional buffer for patients as they realize that their problem is not unique to them, but also help them gain knowledge of how others are dealing with it and enable them to socialize in a *'safe non-judgemental'* group. Often individuals develop emotional bonding with other group members. In many such groups, in-group agenda/rules may be made and followed. Members may decide to chant together, be in touch over social media, play internet/virtual games and, in this and many other ways, be a support to each other.

Now let us see how psychotherapies are combined to help a person with chronic pain. We will revisit the case of Mrs Annu (chapter 3) and see what emerged during the therapy sessions. If you recall, she did not have any major injury but had developed persistent pain and had become hypervigilant. During one of the initial sessions where *ventilation* method was used, this was what she said:

'One day my husband and son sat with me and my daughter-in-law to resolve our differences. They asked both of us to compromise and be friends. My impudent daughter-in-law had the cheek to say that she never quarrelled with me and it was I who started quarrels. She also said that even when I was ill-tempered with her child, she tolerated it and kept quiet. Just see doctor, I have suddenly become the villain in the house. Both my husband and son supported my daughter-in-law rather than me and said that it was I who needed to mend my ways to maintain peace

in our house. Would I not feel insulted and neglected? Do you not agree that my son loves his wife more than his mother?'

These thoughts were dealt in a later session where CBT was the choice of therapy as was described above.

At this juncture, I asked her as to how often she ruminated on these thoughts. She replied, 'All the time.' She further added that since the pain specialist could detect no organic cause for the pain, her family believed that she was faking it. It was only when the constant and persisting pain affected her mobility and functionality that everyone woke up to her suffering. She said, 'I have shown them that the pain is real.' I gently asked her, 'Was proving your point so essential to you?'

'Of course,' she replied defensively. 'I always do. I watch my daughter-in-law and keep tabs of where she goes wrong and then tell my husband and son about it. After all, they should know that she does so many wrong things, too.'

Strategically, I remained silent. After staring at me with rather blazing eyes, she paused to consider what she had just admitted. She suddenly dissolved into tears and sobs racked her body. Once she calmed down, I asked her whom had she been most unkind to. She said it was her daughter-in-law. I shook my head and invited her to think again. 'Perhaps myself,' she said dully. At that I nodded my head. For the first time it had dawned on her that various factors were indirectly affecting her physical health and chronic pain. These included her depression, stubbornness and her anger against her son and daughter-in-law, which also reflected on her grand-daughter.

The upshot of a few joint psychotherapeutic sessions with the entire family was that communication channels, which were hitherto closed with the daughter-in-law, were now opened and forged between them.

It was explained to the family and Mrs Annu that psychological factors had become so enormous that the original physical condition had somehow got overshadowed, and that were now contributing to her chronic pain. *The family now understood Mrs Annu's angst and distress. A combination of medications (antidepressants), dry needling sessions acupuncture and physiotherapy, combined with psychotherapeutic sessions, helped her to recover and she was gradually rehabilitated. Depression, anxiety, hypervigilance and relations with both her son and daughter-in-law improved. In her last follow-up, after six months of intensive intervention, she walked into my chamber all cheerful and holding the hand of her granddaughter.*

Alternative Therapies for Chronic Pain[30]

Acupuncture

Acupuncture is a Traditional Chinese Medicine (TCM) treatment that originated in China more than 2,000 years ago. From its origins in the East, it has spread to Western countries and the rest of the world. Acupuncture is now a reasonable option of treatment for chronic pain in several conditions, such as low back pain, osteoarthritis, headaches, especially migraine, neck pain, fibromyalgia and temporomandibular joint disorders. Recent research has also substantiated the long-lasting effectiveness of acupuncture and endorsed its use for chronic pain.[31]

The theory behind it is that when needles are applied to specific points in the body, the life energy flowing in our body, called Qi, is redirected or invigorated. It has been shown that acupuncture modulates the body's natural painkillers and 'feel good' chemicals such as endorphins and serotonin. This has not only a beneficial effect on pain but also mood and general well-being. It is postulated that acupuncture acts by blocking the neural gates at the spinal cord and prevents pain impulses from reaching the brain (Gate Control Theory). Thus, preventing pain impulses from reaching the brain. Whatever the mechanism of action, acupuncture is definitely an important part of complementary and alternative medicine and can be beneficial in the multidisciplinary integrative rehabilitation of patients with chronic pain, for not only relieving pain but promoting overall well-being.

Homeopathy

Homeopathy is an alternative branch of medicine that treats ailments with minute doses of natural substances. The basic belief is that 'like cures like'. In other words, the cumulative effect of small doses of natural substances would produce similar symptoms of the illness and, thus, trigger the body's natural defences. Though some consider homeopathy more as a placebo, researchers consider it effective in many kinds of acute and chronic pain conditions, namely back pain, musculoskeletal pains, trigeminal neuralgia and headaches. Patients were found to have better reduction in pain and improved quality of life when using homeopathic drugs, as compared to conventional treatment for chronic musculoskeletal conditions.[32]

Ayurveda

Ayurveda is an alternative branch of medicine that originated in India several thousand years ago. It is a holistic treatment that believes in balancing body, mind and spirit. Ayurveda focuses on the five elements of nature, namely fire, earth, air, space and water that make the three energies called 'doshas' in a person. The three doshas—kapha (water and earth), pitta (fire and water) and vata (space and air)—are present in everyone but uniquely differ for each individual. To rectify any ailment, particularly chronic pain, the emphasis is to bring a change in lifestyle along with detoxification (panchakarma) using herbs, massage, change in diet and stress management. Although there is a paucity of creditable research on the efficiency and efficacy of Ayurveda, its usage is highly popular in India, especially for musculoskeletal joint pain.

Spiritual Therapy

Prayer can be considered as a complementary and alternative method of therapy for chronic pain. Prayer is a conversation between a person and a superpower or God. Both prayers and praying act as an emotional buffer to anyone in distress. The importance of prayer lies in the belief system of the person. Those who have strong religious faith find comfort and strength in prayer, especially when they are suffering in pain. Talking or conversing with God as a friend or a parental figure helps in confronting and acknowledging many thoughts and emotions that one may find difficult to confide even in people close to them. Hence, it also has a cathartic value as pent-up emotions get released. However, if God is viewed as punitive parental figure and needs to be appeased, the benefits of prayer are fewer.

Chronic pain patients who have strong faith in God, are encouraged to pray. Prayers and meditation have many similarities, except that while meditation is inward concentration, prayer is an appeal upwards to God. Both decrease stress and anxiety and, additionally, bring serenity and peace to a troubled mind. We saw Rahul's anxiety reducing after his mother asked him to recite some shlokas. Chronic pain research has found that prayers, as a means to cope, are often done not only by patients but also by caregivers.[33]

The Impact of Covid-19 on Treatment of Pain

The Covid-19 pandemic has had a major impact on the treatment of chronic pain. It is a fact that treatment of pain has been declared a fundamental human right,[34] and according to international human rights law, countries have to provide pain treatment medications as part of their core obligations under the right to health. It further states that failure to take reasonable steps to ensure that people who suffer pain have access to adequate pain treatment, may result in the violation of the obligation to protect against cruel, inhuman and degrading treatment.

Yet, during the pandemic, we saw that all medical resources had to be diverted and redistributed to hospitals and ICUs taking care of Covid-19 affected patients. Attendance to most pain clinics dropped drastically and all elective interventional pain management procedures were put in abeyance to prevent the spread of the dreaded virus. This had led to undertreatment of pain, with many patients suffering helplessly.

Besides the undertreatment, inappropriate treatment of pain also posed a hazard during the pandemic. Steroids, in particular, was a double-edged sword. While it had its beneficial effect in certain cases of Covid-19, but by causing immunosuppression it also had a potential to adversely affect the course of the disease. This is also true of opioids, which can affect both innate and acquired immunity. Both these drugs, which are frequently used to treat pain, were either withheld or used cautiously during the pandemic.

In conclusion, we have seen that there is no dearth of medical, physical, psychological and social therapies that are available to help alleviate chronic pain. The skill lies in selecting and incorporating these therapies to maximally help the sufferer. Let us see in the next chapter how Rahul was rehabilitated by integrating various therapies and dealing with his physical, emotional, familial, conjugal and spiritual predicaments.

8

Integrated Rehabilitation Management: A Case Discussion

A comprehensive and integrated multidisciplinary pain rehabilitation programme focuses on the person rather than just the disease. The aim is to improve the wellness of the patient and restore functionality in all spheres of living, be it home, at work or in society. In fact, the WHO defines health as 'a state of complete physical, mental and social well-being and not merely the absence of disease or infirmity'.[1] Similarly, pain also encompasses physical, mental, social and spiritual aspects, which need to be dealt with to restore the total well-being of the person and his or her functionality to the maximum extent.

Rehabilitation for chronic pain encompasses an integrated approach that usually involves multiple specialists, hence, the term multidisciplinary. A team approach is necessary with a shared decision-making process that takes into account inputs of the different healthcare providers who need to address various facets of the problem. These are then integrated and incorporated with the person's and their family members' goals and values. It is, therefore, necessary that all the stakeholders together agree upon realistic goals, so that both physical and mental suffering is reduced, residual function is preserved and, as far as possible, functionality in all its aspects restored. Part of the treatment programme includes the need to focus on the patient and family's disillusionment and disappointment with previous treatments and their outcomes. Most persons who visit pain clinics narrate a long history of umpteen treatment modalities, both traditional and non-traditional, which they had tried time and again without much success. In an integrated pain management rehabilitation programme, the emphasis is not wholly focused on physical pain management alone but is aimed at healing the emotional, behavioural and social problems that maintain and compound the chronic pain and, importantly, helping the patient to come to terms with their residual pain.[2]

A multidisciplinary, integrated pain rehabilitation programme can be lucidly explained with an example of a chronic pain patient with whom we had worked with extensively. We are taking up the case of Rahul (see chapter one) as we had to cope with innumerable aspects of chronic pain while he was under our treatment. These included biological, psychological, familial, occupational and even spiritual issues.

We first began with assessment, both physical and psychological, and then tailored an appropriate treatment based on that.

Physical Assessment

To recapitulate the case history of Rahul, the second accident which he had sustained had caused multiple injuries that left him both physically and psychologically devastated. Besides the fractures in his left thigh and forearm, he had fractured his pelvic bone and dislocated his left shoulder. Unfortunately, he did not get adequate pain relief at that time and that was probably one of the reasons that the acute pain transitioned into chronic pain.

His shoulder muscles had stiffened and there were knots and taut bands in them, which caused myofascial pain. This pain radiated to the back of his head and face. Being in a cast for his fractured leg and the enforced bed rest for fracture of his pelvis had caused stiffness in his lower back, hips and legs. This not only led to physical deconditioning due to prolonged bed-rest-induced disuse atrophy of the muscles, but also resulted in myofascial pain of his back and legs as well. Moreover, being bedridden because of his fractured pelvis had hampered his ambulatory process. The physiotherapy that should have been done early on during the course of rehabilitation, could not be done in a timely manner, which further aggravated matters.

Medical Management

Despite evidence of good healing at the site of his fractures, he still had persistent pain. This pain was predominantly myofascial in origin and was seen as tightening of muscles, taut bands and knots in the muscles of his neck, shoulders, lower back and legs. To relieve the pain, Rahul had been taking over-the-counter anti-inflammatory drugs on a regular basis, with little to no relief. Indeed, myofascial pain responds only temporarily to these drugs and, in some instances, they are not effective at all in relieving this kind of pain. Our primary aim was to wean him away from strong analgesics and substitute them with milder ones, along with muscle relaxants and anti-depressants. The latter helps increase the serotonin and norepinephrine levels and, thus, it not only activates the descending inhibitory pain pathways and relieves pain, but also serves to improve mood and sleep.

Our strategy was to primarily focus on non-drug modalities, rather than just medications. We did so for two reasons. Firstly, his past history of substance abuse precluded excessive use of medications, especially strong analgesics like opioids. Secondly, for Rahul's type of pain (myofascial), a combination of modalities like trigger point injections and dry needling would have least side effects and be more beneficial in the long run.

We started with trigger point injections to release the knots in the muscles and reduce the tender areas. The left shoulder was targeted first, followed by the muscles of his low back and buttock (gluteus muscles). The reason why trigger point injections are given in chronic pain cases, especially when myofascial pain is predominant, is because they help in deactivating the myofascial trigger points by relaxing the taut bands and knots in them. This, in turn, promotes improved blood circulation to the hitherto hypoxic/ischemic area in the affected muscle allowing for removal of metabolic waste products, and, thus, breaks the pain-tension cycle.[3] These injections reduced the tenderness in the myofascial trigger points of his shoulder and buttocks and paved the way for introducing the next modality, dry needling.

Dry needling was incorporated in Rahul's treatment regime to further augment the effect of trigger point injections and relax the taut shoulder, neck and back muscles. One of the mechanisms of action of dry needling is to relax taut muscles. This decreases the barrage of pain impulses proceeding from the periphery (muscles and fascia) to the spinal cord and thence to the brain. This disruption in the pain impulses prevents peripheral and central sensitization of the spinal cord and the brain and decreases the perception of pain.[4] In addition, physiotherapy interventions, discussed in more detail later on, were also initiated alongside to further supplement the effects of the trigger point injections and dry needling. For the first two months, Rahul received dry needling sessions twice a week and thereafter once a week. In all, over a period of three months, twenty dry needling sessions were done.

During the dry needling sessions, we also stimulated acupuncture points in his shoulders, arms, low back and legs. Since the same type of needles are used for both dry needling and acupuncture, it made this task relatively easy. The reason for adding acupuncture with dry needling was that stimulating the myofascial trigger points with acupuncture is known to relieve myofascial pain and irritability. Moreover, acupuncture therapy—when combined with medical therapy—has been found to be beneficial in treating chronic pain associated with depression, as heavy doses of antidepressants alone may be associated with serious drug-related side effects.[5] We found the combination of dry needling and acupuncture beneficial for Rahul.

Physical Therapy

The interventions performed in the Pain Clinic were further coordinated with daily physiotherapy to further boost the effect of the pain interventions. The modalities used included transcutaneous electrical nerve stimulation (TENS), interferential therapy (IFT) and low-level laser therapy (cold laser therapy). These were combined with active exercises, which included strengthening, stretching, conditioning, myofascial release along with postural correction. These techniques helped in reversing the physical deconditioning that had set in Rahul, helped relax the muscles that had stiffened and, at the same time, strengthened the weak muscles. As mentioned above, dry needling combined with stretching was particularly beneficial for Rahul because it inactivated the painful trigger points in muscles and reduced discomfort while doing the active stretching.[6]

A few sessions were devoted to myofascial release using massage therapies that focused on releasing tightness and shortness of the muscles of his shoulders and low back. This further improved Rahul's flexibility and the range of movement of his shoulder and arm. With reduced pain and better mobility, his fatigue and depression also decreased, thereby increasing his functionality. Now Rahul reported that he could lift his son without wincing in pain, and that brought down his anxiety and hypervigilance whenever his son was around him.

But just as you cannot clap with one hand alone, medical management along with interventional pain management and physical therapy alone were not sufficient to treat Rahul's chronic pain problem as it had serious underlying psychological ramifications as well. In an integrated pain management programme, the psychological, social and spiritual angst in Rahul also had to be addressed. So, let us see how we initiated psychological therapy side by side, by first assessing his psychological issues.

Psychological Assessment

Personality test (Eysenck Personality Questionnaire-Revised {EPQR}) revealed high scores on psychoticism and extraversion. This indicated that he had personality traits such as aggressiveness, manipulation, tough-mindedness, risk-taking, irresponsibility and impulsivity. Since the neuroticism score was low and extraversion score was high, he fitted in the 'stable extravert' category with sanguine qualities such as being outgoing, talkative, responsive, easy-going, lively and carefree and having leadership qualities.

The clinical tests indicated moderate depression, very high survivor's guilt and guilt also related to lack of achievement, disappointment in his relationship with his wife, high anxiety related to his pain, strong fears of disability and sleep disturbance.

On the Coping Scale he had scored very high on mental and behavioural disengagement and use of emotional support from his mother. Although he showed a strong desire to use substances to cope with his pain, yet he had resisted it.

Based on his assessment, we explained to Rahul that various unresolved psychological issues were further restricting his ability to optimize his functionality and needed to be tackled for relief from chronic pain.

Since rapport was already established on his very first visit, I now needed to focus on what required urgent attention. Like most patients, Rahul, too, was overwhelmed with feelings of hopelessness and helplessness. He needed reassurance and it became my first and foremost task to reassure him that chronic pain is fairly common, but with the right multidisciplinary approach, there is likely to be a light at the end of the tunnel.

Initiating Psychotherapy

Once again, I emphasized to Rahul the importance of physical activity, exercise, nutrition and reconditioning of the body and mind in promoting healing. I also provided some information on neuro-anatomy and neurophysiology. While using the reassurance technique of supportive psychotherapy, some of the information was repeated to reiterate various facets of chronic pain that included the contribution of physiological, psychological and behavioural factors. Now that his confidence in the team treating him was established and we had the knowledge of his psychological profile, we began our sessions.

The initial sessions were devoted to the ventilation method because the need to talk about his friends and the accident were predominant in his mind. Since no one had really volunteered information about the fate of his friends, he had guessed that perhaps something very serious had occurred. As conversation was always manoeuvred away from the accident, one day he had accosted his wife to tell him the truth. Reminiscing about that day he said, 'I remember being shocked with disbelief on hearing what had happened that fateful day. I felt searing anger within myself with such severe pain in my chest that I felt I could not breathe. I could hear some voices from a distance but could not comprehend anything as my mind felt completely blank. I do not remember what was done to me but after sometime I slept. Oh! The oblivion was a relief.' His face was contorted with grief and his hands were trembling even as he spoke; it was obvious that he was deeply affected by it. It was an effort for him to hold back his tears.

In the next session he described his feelings, sense of confusion, feeling emotionally drained and anger towards God (spiritual pain). He appeared frustrated at so many unanswered questions. He said, 'My belief in God was limited to pujas at home where I was compelled to participate. However, for the first time I prayed in earnest for forgiveness. Had I not suggested that race, all my friends would have been alive today, and Ravi would have been enjoying a happy family life with his wife and daughter. Oh doctor! I feel so guilty. Why was I, a useless and unworthy person, spared?' The anguish and guilt were palpably present.

In the third session he spoke about having nightmares where he would hear the sound of wheels crunching so loudly that he would wake up breathless and sweating. He confessed that on such nights he had a strong desire to resort to alcohol to drown the sounds and guilt he felt. Though he had resisted use of substances until now, I saw that it was definitely an area that needed resolution.

Dealing with guilt

It was obvious that Rahul was suffering from *survivor's guilt*. Since this was troubling him so much, the need to address it first was strongly indicated. So CBT was introduced in the fourth session. The process started with first analysing the guilt he felt. The guilt was mainly related to two thoughts, namely suggesting the race and surviving it. The first thought was targeted as follows:

R: *If I had not suggested the race everyone would have been alive and well.*

T: *Tell me more about what led to this suggestion.*

R: Well, you see doctor, Subodh (a friend who had died in the accident) had said that as we were planning to lead a straitjacketed life from then on, we should live it up that night. (He paused while reflecting).

T: Then… (prompting)

R: We all unanimously agreed with his suggestion. Everyone came up with different ideas on how to make the evening memorable. It was then that I remembered that on the last day of our college (we were all college friends), we had done a motorbike race for the same reason, something to remember in our old age. Since we wanted to remember that momentous day, too, in a similar way, the idea was endorsed by all.

T: I'm hearing you say that though you proposed the idea, it was supported wholeheartedly by all.

R: Yes, that is true.

T: Once again to clarify, I take it that it was a unanimous decision and made for sentimental reasons. Now would you like to re-evaluate the responsibility of the decision?

R: Are you saying this to make me feel better?

T: (Smiling) It is good if you feel better. But objectively speaking, don't you think the onus of the decision lies with everyone? You have used the word endorsed, which indicates that everyone gave their consent for the race.

R: Yes. In fact, we were betting too. We bet that whoever wins the race, would foot the bill for the tea. We all were laughing uproariously because in our student days our pockets were always empty and everyone would be borrowing from the other. Payment for our outings was always an issue despite us getting more than enough from our parents.

T: Would you like to rethink this thought about being responsible for the race?

R: *Doc, it is nice of you to shift the blame, but it is not decent to blame dead people.*

T: *Rahul, at the moment we are being objective and unsentimental. We are not blaming anyone in particular because, as you clearly have stated, it was a collective decision.*

R: *Yes, it was (Became silent and seemed to be contemplating).*

T: *(Remained silent too)*

R: *(Heaving a sigh) I believe what you say is correct. I cannot absolutely absolve myself but, yes, we all had decided together to have a race.*

The session was terminated soon after and homework was given to reflect what happened during the session and to write down his thoughts and feelings about it.

In a similar fashion, his guilt about surviving the accident was also tackled. Another aspect that was discussed in the sessions was that it was the other car that had lost control first and rammed into Rahul's car. It was purely a case of accident.

CBT was not the only method used. Many other ways were also used for making him get over the survivor's guilt. As the anniversary of the accident was drawing close, a suggestion was made about visiting the parents of his late friends. Rahul himself came up with the idea of holding a prayer meeting for his friends and inviting their families for it. This helped him to grieve openly for his friends for the first time. He felt relieved, too, as the parents of his deceased friends were sympathetic towards him and no word of blame was laid on him. Subodh's father was tearful and said that his son had always been a high-spirited person who would have preferred death to leading a life with disability.

Rahul's guilt was maximally with regard to Ravi who was being nursed at home in a vegetative state. Rahul did not have the heart to face him and repeatedly gave the excuse that since his friend would not recognize him anyway, there was no point in seeing him. This distorted thought was then challenged. He did acknowledge that one visited the sick for one's own satisfaction of their welfare. It was also pointed out that some kind of resolution needed to take place vis-à-vis this friend, too, so that he could find peace. During the session he was reminded of his resolve to be a father figure to Ravi's daughter who was by then fifteen months old. If he did not meet the child, what role was he likely to play in her life?

A significant incident happened during his visit to Ravi's home. Ravi's wife was keen to know exactly what had happened on that fateful evening. She was overwhelmed when she heard of Ravi's decision to choose her and their daughter, over his friends and the flamboyant and irresponsible life he was leading. She then confided in Rahul and his wife that she had been extremely angry with Ravi and had often thought of going back to her parents' house rather than be his caregiver for life. In fact, while narrating this incident to me, Rahul contemplatively said that perhaps God had saved him so that he could bring solace to Ravi's wife. The confession of anger by Ravi's wife resonated with Rahul's wife, too, and it forged a strong bond of friendship between the two women.

Introduction of adjuvant methods

Other supportive psychotherapeutic methods were now added. Rahul was fond of music and had, as a child, learnt to play the keyboard. He was now encouraged to practice it and teach his son too. He voluntarily took up art and dance movement therapy, scheduling it on alternative days. This helped him to distract his mind. Dance movement therapy became an adjunct to physiotherapy as his mobility increased. An added advantage was that he re-learned to socialize and made new friends in these classes.

Rahul was not very easy to work with. His motivation levels would fluctuate and, on some days, he would come for the sessions in an extremely irritable mood. These mood fluctuations had to be tackled, too, as resistance to therapy hampers the therapeutic process. On such occasions, he would remark that one of the reasons for his irritability was an increase in pain. However, during an individual psychotherapeutic session it transpired that he was getting annoyed by the constant presence of his family members around him and even expressed it as, 'I don't need babysitters.'

It was perhaps also the first time since their marriage that he was spending quality time with his wife and actually getting to know her. But due to the constant presence of one or the other family member around him, he barely got an opportunity to be alone with her. At this stage of the rehabilitation we had to incorporate sessions initially with his family, which included his parents and extended family, and later with his spouse.

Dealing with family and couple issues: Three sessions were devoted to family therapy. In the first session the entire extended family was present. Their roles were discussed regarding providing support to Rahul and his wife. It was then decided that since Rahul was improving there was no need to be oversolicitous and hover over him all the time. The timings were so arranged that the aunts could attend to their office work and by rotation be at home to help.

In the second session only his parents were present. Rahul had shown a leaning towards his mother for support, which was encouraged at that point in time. He said he had realized that his mother was a down-to-earth person and trusted her more than others to help his wife to bring up their son. In a gainful insight he even said, 'If perhaps my mother had the sole charge in bringing me up, I may not have been sitting here today. I may not have grown up wild and irresponsible.'

A third session was devoted to Rahul, his wife and mother. Rahul expressed his wish to his wife that he was keen to let his mother guide and participate in the upbringing of their son. His wife readily agreed to this suggestion. In fact, she was rather relieved and confessed that the only person she actually trusted for her son's upbringing was her mother-in-law. She further added that she became a devoted mother to her son simply because her role as a wife was limited due to Rahul's flamboyant lifestyle. And since the accident, everyone had literally pushed her aside to look after him. As many major decisions were taken by the family and openly communicated, the family was now expected to understand their respective roles and proactively adhere to them.

Rahul's treatment still remained incomplete. His relationship with his wife had to be sorted out and improved. We then began the couple therapy. Many issues were dealt with. These related predominantly to lack of open communication between them, earlier disagreements about Rahul's lifestyle, absence of intimacy and the current fear of his wife that once well, he might revert to his old lifestyle.

A significant agenda that required a special session, and was the core of the anger that his wife harboured against him, was the placement of the burden of his irresponsible behaviour on her by the extended family. On hearing this, Rahul was initially shocked, then enraged. However, he was helped to work through his emotions before leaving my chamber, as at this point there was no question of setting off recriminations amongst the family members. However, that night he again experienced severe pain and was unable to sleep.

The next day he telephoned asking for another session. Instead of a complete session he was asked to meet me for a short duration. I found him emotionally charged again, and he was literally squirming in his chair trying to make himself more comfortable. When I asked him the reason for this restlessness, he replied that he was in pain. The reason for the visit was that he was once again feeling guilty, this time for the blame being meted out to his wife for his deeds. Almost magically, he had an insight and asked whether his being emotionally agitated could be the reason for his pain. When I nodded my head, he visibly tried to control himself. It was apparent that emotional regulation was yet to take place.

By now a fair progress had been made in several domains. Rahul was beginning to gain insight into his own behaviour, a process of self-revelation. After the initial seven to eight psychotherapeutic sessions in combination with pain interventions and physical therapy, there was a significant reduction in pain and improvement in mood. He reported feeling less depressed and anxious. Moreover, during the psychotherapeutic sessions, catharsis had taken place for both Rahul and his wife, and the angst and anger that she carried against him were resolved to a large extent.

Also, since the time he had met his friends' parents, a sense of relief had set in, further reducing his guilt feelings. His anxiety levels had noticeably reduced and he felt a new-found hope that his pain would be largely relieved and his functionality would improve. Despite these positive developments, he also came to the stark realization that he would have to live with some residual pain. His individual psychotherapy sessions needed to be continued as he had to still learn to cope with adversity, not resort to substance use as a coping mechanism; learn to live with his pain and yet work towards his cherished goals.

Increasing coping skills: As we approached the fifteenth session, an eclectic approach was decided upon primarily using behaviour therapy, problem-solving methods to increase coping mechanisms and anger and stress management. Although Rahul had decided to turn over a new leaf and had left alcohol and drugs after the accident, yet he was often tempted to revert under conditions of intolerable pain, stress and guilt. We knew, historically, how physiotherapy had been replaced by alcohol and drugs at the behest of his friends. As we were not keen on that repeating, it was an issue that had to be dealt with urgently. From our experience we know that many patients suffering from chronic pain are victims of substance use disorder (SUD) or, put in simpler terms, drug addiction.

At this juncture, learning of coping mechanisms was facilitated so that his desire for alcohol in times of adversity was reduced. Two persons were chosen to help him out, his wife and mother. Rahul was encouraged to talk and communicate his feelings and frustrations to them, instead of thinking of taking alcohol as an alternative. The increased communication was found helpful by him. Simultaneously, problem-solving strategies were taught. It was explained to him that since problems were unavoidable, instead of reacting to them it was prudent to mindfully and deliberately strategize behaviours to come up with healthy solutions. This process involves brainstorming and coming up with several solutions, picking the most advantageous one, implementing it and seeing the outcomes. If this was successful, to continue with the solution, but if not, then to go back to the other solutions and pick the second best and follow the same process. This way any and many kinds of problems could be dealt with, without getting emotionally upset.

Since Rahul was a reactive person, emotional regulation skills also had to be taught to him. Instead of reacting negatively to adversity and frustrations, he was encouraged to control and moderate his reactions. Whenever negative emotions arose, he needed to process them and let them go. Holding on to negative emotions, as happened when he was angry with his extended family, would only bring back pain and increase his desire for alcohol. Additionally, he needed to be mindful of replacing negative thoughts with positive ones.

As Rahul was prone to anger and could get upset easily, some simple anger management techniques were taught to him. Here both progressive muscular relaxation and simple yoga exercises were introduced. He was encouraged to seek help from a trained yoga instructor who would help him at home. The simple preliminary steps of mindfulness meditation were initiated, too, to help him remain calm. All the three methods helped him remain relaxed and a lot more serene.

During one of the sessions, he mentioned that his mother had insisted that he recite some shlokas in the morning. When asked how he felt about praying he replied rather shyly that he felt a lot of comfort when he did recite those shlokas. Since praying was helping him emotionally, he was encouraged to continue doing so. I explained that spirituality brings hope, comfort, solace and self-accountability, which empowers a person. It would give him strength to say no to alcohol too.

As Rahul's pain began subsiding and resolutions to many intra-relationship and inter-relationship conflicts had taken place, he was now encouraged to attend office daily for two hours. Slowly, with further improvement, the hours spent in the office were increased. Vocational rehabilitation is an important aspect of rehabilitation of patients with chronic pain. It involves a return to work and is usually initiated in the latter part of the rehabilitation programme, after the initial improvement in physical and psychological functioning. Some, however, believe that vocational counselling and training should be initiated as early as possible in the programme.

At this point of time, we clinicians met to review Rahul's progress and, if possible, to start fading out sessions with him. It had been almost four months of intensive work with him and his family. Dr Abraham, the Pain Clinic head, after two months of dry needling/ acupuncture sessions twice a week, had reduced the dry needling sessions to once a week as there was a significant improvement in pain. She had gradually weaned him off the analgesics and muscle relaxants, too, and he was only taking a minimal dose of antidepressant drugs by then. After the initial intensive physiotherapy sessions for two months, the physiotherapist reported that Rahul no longer needed to come to the centre anymore and he could do the exercises meticulously at home on a daily basis. He had learnt those adequately and there was no need for daily supervision.

Dr Prakash added that Rahul had himself reported reduction in his chronic pain and feelings of depression, anxiety and guilt. Since he was beginning to manage himself physically, mentally and occupationally, the psychotherapy sessions also needed to be terminated. We all agreed that an integrated approach combining drug and non-drug therapies—which included pain interventions, physical therapy, complementary and alternative medicine, psychotherapy, family therapy and occupational therapy—was indeed proving beneficial for Rahul. We all parted on that optimistic note.

In the last session of psychotherapy, Rahul was asked to evaluate his four-month-long journey with us. He gravely told me that he now felt emotionally stable, more responsible, had purpose in life and found strength within himself. He was contented that his wife was no longer a stranger but was a warm, loving and caring person. He acknowledged that the relationship with his wife and family were no longer the enmeshed kind, but instead, supportive, compassionate and encouraging. Now that his pain had reduced, his anxiety related to being hurt by the playful behaviour of his son had lessened and he found himself spending more time playing with his child. His parting words were, 'I need to thank you all for making me feel wholesome once again. I have learnt that chronic pain is a complex mind-body game in which somewhere the mind also has to be trained to control the body pain.'

To summarize, when Rahul had come to us he had been experiencing pain which was rather complex in nature. Physically he was experiencing post-traumatic myofascial pain, psychologically he was suffering from depression, anxiety and guilt feelings, socially he was isolated from friends and colleagues and had enmeshed relationship with family members, occupationally he was not involved in any constructive work and spiritually he considered pain as punishment and penance for his wrongdoings. During the rehabilitation programme, all these issues were dealt with one by one, some with more success than the others. Nonetheless, Rahul did benefit from this integrated, multidisciplinary approach, which we had worked out for him, in tandem with him, his family and also with each other. Like well-oiled machinery, the success of the multidisciplinary approach depended a lot on Rahul's cooperation and high motivation levels, along with a seamless inter-disciplinary understanding and awareness amongst the treating clinicians.

It must be appreciated that every individual is unique. This individuality determines the thoughts, emotions and behaviours of the person, making it distinctive, complex and dynamic. Each individual differs in their ability to understand and realize the extent to which the trilogy of their own cognitions, affect and behaviours influences their experience with chronic pain. Though it can be said that negative emotions—particularly sadness, anger, anxiety and guilt and unresolved conflicts—have a bearing on a person's life, they have a greater effect on chronic pain patients. The insight into their exceptional set of problems and the realization that mind and body are two sides of the same coin is of considerable essence. When all these factors form a favourable constellation, the efficacy of the treatment programme is better guaranteed.

From the clinicians' side, time needs to be expended and efforts put in to glean as much information as possible from the patient and the family to earmark the areas that need rectification. Only then can the multimodal techniques be judicially and strategically utilized to reduce pain, whether it is emotional, physical, social or sometimes spiritual too. The objective of rehabilitation in chronic pain patients is to make them, as far as possible, pain-free, functional, self-reliant and emotionally stable. The key to their life has to be firmly handed back to them.

Dear readers, you must have gathered that chronic pain patients need holistic treatment where every aspect that has gone awry needs to be addressed, with emphasis on strengthening of the mind to manage chronic pain.

As has been aptly said,

'If I were somebody dealing with chronic pain, I would see it as a challenge to manage my mind; even knowing that the effect of my thoughts is not only affecting my experience, but it is absolutely affecting my state of health.'

—Cheryl Richardson

Acknowledgements

A book for an author is like a child that needs to be nourished in order to thrive healthily. Each child, while growing up, faces unusual and, at times, difficult circumstances. This child of ours grew up in the unprecedented times of the Covid-19 pandemic. It saw the lockdown, untold miseries and a galore of calamities. During this time, we both were heavily engaged, professionally and personally, and each wrote the book either late at night or in the wee hours of the morning. While winding up the book, our families and us had a brush with Covid-19, its accompanying anxiety, uncertainty and, even, fear. That was very distracting, to put it mildly, and made it rather difficult for us to concentrate on the task of finishing the book. Suffice to say, by the grace of God and the help rendered by our family, friends and well-wishers saw us through those troubled times and we managed to accomplish our target.

We owe our gratitude first and foremost to our patients who, wittingly or unwittingly, allowed us to peep into their lives and thereby form the crux of this book. With no holds barred, sharing of experiences by the patients, enabled us to gain insight into the minds and behaviours that precipitate and maintain chronicity of pain. We wish to thank all of them. The names used in the book are fictitious, but the stories are true.

Acknowledgements

We wish to thank our respective doctors who pulled us and our families out of the quagmire of Covid-19 infection and its after-effects. Vandana wishes to thank Dr Jyoti Jain, Dr Anurag Jain, Dr Savyasachi Saxena and Dr C. Balakrishnan for being prompt in giving medications and guidance to combat the disease in home quarantine.

Mary wishes to thank Dr Rahul Nagpal, Dr Savita Nagpal, Dr Mughda Tapdiya and Mrs Hema Siddhartha Chand for the unstinted support they offered so unhesitatingly to her family during the pandemic.

We owe gratitude to our publisher HarperCollins India for believing in us and giving us another opportunity to bring a sequel to our earlier book, *Conquering Pain: How to Prevent it, Treat it and Lead a Better Life*.

No author can overlook the silent, but vociferous contribution of their family members. Without their support, constructive criticism and giving space to us to write, this book would not have seen the light of the day. Vandana wishes to thank her husband, Navin Prakash, two lovely and cherished daughters, Shreya and Srishti, sister, Ranjana Sharma, and her nephew, Abhijit. Forever in her heart are the images of her parents, Shakuntala and Prahlad Narain Varma, who, though gathered in the bosom of Our Lord, continue to inspire her.

Mary also wishes to thank her husband, Abraham Punnose, devoted sons, Ashish and Nishant, talented and doting daughters-in-law, Madhavi and Tania, loving and adorable grandchildren, Advait, Aditi and little Daniel, and her late dear parents and parents-in-law, for always encouraging and enabling her to reach out to people suffering in pain. She especially wishes to thank the eminent pain specialist, Dr Lakshmi Vas, for always being her friend, philosopher and guide in her journey of treating patients in pain.

Last and not the least, there are so many persons who directly or indirectly have helped us in numerous ways while we wrote the book. A special thanks to all of them.

Glossary

1. **Adjuvant analgesics:** medication that is not primarily a pain-relieving drug, but can alleviate pain when given in conjunction with other pain-relieving drugs. Some examples are anticonvulsant drugs, antidepressant drugs, steroids and muscle relaxants.
2. **Agoraphobia:** is an anxiety disorder that involves an extreme and irrational fear of being unable to escape a difficult or embarrassing situation resulting in panic-like states or other incapacitating symptoms.
3. **Allodynia:** a phenomenon where even a non-painful stimulus like touching the skin could cause pain. It is a characteristic feature of neuropathic pain.
4. **Behavioural theories:** these theories are based on learning principles of objective and observable behaviours and are acquired through conditioning.
5. **Biofeedback:** a behavioural therapy method used for controlling some of the functions of the body like heart rate, muscle tone and pain perception. This technique involves being connected to electrical sensors that give feedback/information about one's body.

6. **Central sensitization:** a phenomenon where the neurons in the spinal cord and brain are hyper-excitable, which leads to an enhanced pain experience as seen in chronic pain.

7. **Chronic Regional Pain Syndrome (CRPS):** a chronic neuropathic pain condition which affects a limb (arms or legs), and occurs due to malfunctioning of the peripheral nerves or the central nervous system. It is characterized by pain which is burning in nature, increased sensitivity to touch, swelling and it also may be accompanied by a change in the colour and temperature of the skin.

8. **Cognitive Behavioural Therapy (CBT):** this therapy treats problems with the assumption that dysfunctional thoughts and emotions can be rectified by rationally modifying them.

9. **Dysthymia:** a low level of depression that has lasted for more than two years.

10. **Epidural block:** a local anaesthetic administered to the area outside the tough lining of the spinal cord, the dura mater, which causes numbing of the spinal nerves and consequently relief of pain.

11. **Inflammatory mediators:** substances that are released at the site of injury or inflammation which cause pain. They include substance P, histamine, serotonin, bradykinin and prostaglandins.

12. **Muscle shortening:** persistent state of contraction of a skeletal or voluntary muscle of the body, which leads to a tightness or spasm of the muscle along with pain and tenderness. Muscle shortening is an important cause of myofascial pain.

13. **Myofascial Pain/Myofascial Pain Syndrome:** pain originating from the muscle and its surrounding covering or fascia. It is

characterized by tender points called *myofascial trigger points* and is often referred to a remote region that is specific for a particular muscle.

14. **Neuralgia:** an intense, shooting or electric type of painful sensation along a nerve that is usually intermittent. It may be due to irritation to the nerve or damage to it resulting in its malfunctioning. It is a type of neuropathic pain.

15. **Neuropathic pain:** pain as a result of a disease or lesion in the somatosensory nervous system. Examples are compression of nerve due to degenerated spine, post-herpetic neuralgia (damage to nerve caused by a virus), diabetic neuropathy, trigeminal neuralgia (compression of the trigeminal nerve by an aberrant blood vessel).

16. **Nociceptor:** 'nocere'—to do harm, 'receptor'—a group of cells that receive a stimulus. Nociceptor is a sensor that receives a stimulus which can cause harm or, in other words, a pain sensor.

17. **Nociceptive pain:** pain as a result of tissue damage, which is transmitted to the central nervous system for perception by a normally functioning nervous system.

18. **Peripheral neuropathy:** damage or disease of the peripheral nerves that transmit messages to and from the brain and spinal cord. It results in impairment of sensations, movement and gland or organ function depending on the nerve that is affected. The most common cause of peripheral neuropathy is long-standing diabetes.

19. **Peripheral sensitization:** an increased firing of the pain impulse from the periphery due to release of certain chemicals at the site of tissue damage, which leads to an increased pain experience.

20. **Secondary gains:** the advantages that occur secondary to the real or stated illness itself.

21. **Sciatica:** pain in the low back region, hip and radiating down the leg. It is usually due to compression of the sciatic nerve, which is a large nerve that supplies the lower limbs. The usual causes for nerve compression are herniated intervertebral disc or degenerative changes in the lower spine.

Notes

Scan this QR code to access the detailed notes

Index

abuse, 12, 150; alcohol, 90–91; physical, 36, 59–60; sexual, 36, 50, 60, 75; substance, 22, 49, 77, 108, 191
acceptance and commitment therapy (ACT), 62–66, 173–176
activities of daily living (ADL), 55
acute pain, xiii, 15, 21, 33, 41. See also Chronic pain; defined, 18; duration of, 20; impact of, 20; pain in patients with chronic pain, 19
adult chronic pain, 50
affective vulnerability and chronic pain measures: Beck's Anxiety Inventory, 132; Beck's Depression Inventory, 131; Center for Epidemiological Studies-Depression (CES-D), 132; Depression and Anxiety Stress Scale (DASS), 131–132; Penn's State Worry Questionnaire (PSWQ), 132; Positive and Negative Affect Scale (PANAS), 133; State Trait Anger Expression Inventory (STAXI), 132–133; State Trait Anxiety Inventory (STAI), 132

Algea, 43
algos, 43
allodynia pain, 37–38
alternative therapies for chronic pain: acupuncture, 185–186; Ayurveda, 186; homeopathy, 186; spiritual therapy, 187
Alzheimer's disease, 18
anger, 10, 22, 38, 42, 56–58, 91; expressed, 47, 61; unexpressed, 47
antidepressants, 49, 72, 97, 101, 152, 161, 185, 193, 204

217

anxiety, 6, 10–11, 13–14, 18, 75, 77, 131, 135, 139, 144–145, 149, 165, 167–169, 173, 177–179, 185, 187; -provoking thoughts, 12; behaviour therapy use to reduce, 168; emotional mood, 49–50; pervasive, 103; sensitivity, 59–60
arthralgia, 43
arthritis, 20, 22, 42, 84, 85, 91, 94, 98, 150, 154, 164, 168; osteoarthritis, 33, 39, 88, 98–100, 156–157, 161, 185; rheumatoid, 39, 66, 85, 110, 163
assessment in chronic pain: barriers to, 140–141; in elderly with or without dementia, 139; patients history, 125–126; physical examination of, 141–142; PQRST, 126–127; psychosocial, 130; to conduct investigations, 142–143; tools used for, 127–128; (multidimensional, 129; undimensional, 128); West Haven Yale Multidimensional Pain Inventory (WHYMPI), 129–130
autogenic training, 166

brain fog, 103

behaviour therapies for mind treatment: promotion of relaxation, 165–168; reduction in anxiety, 168; stress inoculation therapy (SIT) (see Stress inoculation therapy (SIT))
behavioural changes, 11, 38, 139
belief role in treatment programme: beliefs in pain control questionnaire (BPCQ), 133; coping strategies questionnaire (CSQ), 134; pain catastrophizing scale (PCS), 134; pain self-efficacy questionnaire (PSEQ), 134
biofeedback, 166–167
Brief Pain Inventory, 129

cancer pain, 21, 85, 108–109, 142, 148–152
caregiver stress syndrome, 117
Cartesian dualism (or substance dualism), 43
central sensitization syndromes, 9–10, 31, 33–40
chemotherapy-induced peripheral neuropathy (CIPN), 85
chronic pain, xiii, xv–xvi, 6–8, 10, 58, 67–69, 125, 144. See also Acute pain; affects/impacts on mind

Index

and body, 13, 50, 95–97; (cardiovascular system, 100; caregivers, 117–118; change in interpersonal relations, 116–117; couple relationship, 115–116; expressed emotions by family, 118–121; fatigue and stiffness, 99; fear, 109; frustration and angry towards others, 108–109; gastrointestinal system, 101; immune system, 101–102; insomnia sleep disorder, 110–111; loneliness and isolation, 109–110; lowered self-esteem, 112–113; on cognitive functions, 103–107; on locomotor system, 97–98; on nervous system, 98–99; physical and emotional fatigue, 110; psychological impact, 102–103; sexual difficulties, 112; shameful feelings, 107–108; sick role development, 113–115; social guilt, 107–108; social relationships, 121–122); Cartesian model, 23–24; central sensitization hallmark of, 37; changes, 12; chronic primary pain, 21; chronic secondary pain, 21–22; cognitive processes in, 60–62; conditions in, 31–32; (brain and central sensitization, 35–37; changes at injury site, 32–33; changes in pain modulation, 37–39; changes in spinal cord and central sensitization, 33–35; run in families, 73); duration of, 20; fear of dependency, 20–21; management of (see Management of chronic pain); mental deconditioning, 11–12; multi-dimensional, 13; multidisciplinary approach, 13; pain is predominant symptom, 22; physical deconditioning, 11; potent stressor, 11; psychological factors, 49; recovery in, 144; sick role, development of, 18; source of righting, 50; using biopsychosocial model, xiv, 8–9; worldwide prevalence of, 21

chronic pain syndrome. *See also* Chronic pain: conditions, 22; defined, 19; psychological symptoms in, 22–23

chronic regional pain syndrome, 37–39

cognitive behaviour therapy (CBT), 161, 196, 198; aims of, 169; automatic negative thoughts (ANTs), 170–173;

distorted thoughts and pain-related cognitions, 169–170; to find distorted thoughts and pain-related cognitions, 169–170 ; acceptance and commitment therapy (ACT) (see Acceptance and commitment therapy (ACT))

comorbid symptoms and chronic pain: Multidimensional Fatigue Inventory (MFI), 131; Multiple Abilities Symptom Questionnaire (MASQ), 130–131; Pittsburgh Sleep Quality Index (PSQI), 131

Covid-19 pandemic, xvi; and impact on pain treatment, 187–188; and impact on physical and mental health, 93–94

depression, 6, 10, 12–14, 18, 22, 30, 37, 40, 42, 46–47, 49, 58, 76–77, 131; associated, 39; post, 36; postpartum, 36

diabetic neuropathy, 82, 142

diathesis-stress model, 57–60

disability, xi, xvi, 7, 12–13, 21, 47, 51, 58–59, 61, 66–67, 79, 89, 91, 102, 104, 106–107, 118–119, 121–122, 124, 126, 130, 161, 177, 182. See also Chronic pain; disease in itself, 19; fear of, 109–110, 194; impact on functionality of person, 56; intellectual, 18; limitations due to, 13; restrictions forced by, 56

distress/distressed/distressful, xiv, 4, 13, 20–21, 31, 47, 50, 57–58, 63–64, 75–76, 78, 83, 102, 112, 120, 144, 166, 176, 178, 185, 187; chronic abdominal pain cause, 85; emotional, 38, 73, 146, 174; feelings, 62; mental, 94; natural, 12

disturbances in cognitive functioning, 38

double aspectism, 44

Douleur Neuropathique (DN4), 130

drug addiction, 203

dysfunctional pain, 20. See also Chronic pain

dysthymia, 22, 77, 87, 104

Emergentism, 44

emotional pain, 9, 64

employment and chronic pain, 124; disclosure about pain, 122; empathetic employer, impact of, 123; factors influence, 122–123

Epiphenomenalism, 44

fear avoidance, 11, 37

fear-avoidance theory, 55–57

Index

fibromyalgia, 21–22, 35–40, 71–72, 74–75, 77, 86–88, 90, 103, 111, 144–145
FLACC scale, 128
functional MRI, 45, 111

gate control theory of pain of (Ronald Melzack and Patrick Wall), 25, 29–30

hyperalgesia pain, 38

inflammatory mediators, 24, 32, 89
injury, 5, 9–10, 12, 14–20, 25, 37; physical, 42, 68; re-, 56; spinal cord, 39; tissue, 21–24, 31–32, 41
integrated multidisciplinary pain rehabilitation programme: adjuvant methods, 199–200; aims of, 189–190; family therapy, 200–202; methods to learn with guilt, 196–199; physical assessment, 190–191; (medical management, 191–193; physical therapy, 193–194); psychological assessment, 194–195; supportive psychotherapy, 195–196; team approach, importance of, 189; to increase coping skills, 202–207; treatment programme, 190

integrative behavioural couple therapy (IBCT), 182
interactionism theory of, 44

Jacobson's Progressive Muscular Relaxation (JPMR), 165

kinesiophobia, 11

Leeds Assessment of Neuropathic Symptoms and Signs (LANSS), 130
lifestyle factors and pain, 87; bad posture, 89; lack of physical activity and exercise, 88; obesity, 88–89; sleep disturbance, 89–90; stress, 90; substance-use disorders, 90–91

management and cure of chronic pain, 146–147; basic and advanced interventions, 153–159; commonly administered analgesics, 150–151; multidisciplinary rehabilitation (see Multidisciplinary rehabilitation); pharmacological therapy, 148–150
McCafferty, Margo, 17
McGill's Pain Questionnaire (MPQ), 129

meditation, 47, 167, 177, 187, 204
mental disorders influencing chronic pain: bodily distress disorder, 79; employment status and occupation, 86–87; joint inflammation or arthritis, 84–85; medical comorbidities, 81; muscle disorders, 84–85; neurological conditions, 81–82; personality characteristics and disorders, 79–80; spine comorbidities, 82–84
mind and chronic pain: biological factors, 49
mind-body: dualism, 43–44; interaction, 51–55; phenomena, 45
modifiable risk factors and chronic pain, 69–70; agoraphobia, 77–79; anxiety, 77; depression, 76–77; generalized anxiety disorder (GAD), 77–78; mental health, 76; pain, 75–76; panic attacks, 78
multidisciplinary rehabilitation: treatment goals and psycho-education, 147–148
muscles, 23–24, 90–92, 191–193; activity, 48; atrophy, 102; contraction, 166; disorder, 84–85; relax, 49; relaxants, 204; shortening, 97–98; spasms, 8, 102, 149, 154; tensing/tensed, 49, 165, 168; wasting, 100; weakness, 102
myalgia, 43
myofascial pain syndrome (MPS), 84, 98

neuralgia, 22, 31, 38, 43, 70, 154, 157, 186
neurological illness, 31, 39, 81
neuropathic pain, 35, 70, 81, 85, 88, 91, 98, 127–130, 142, 152–154, 157–158, 164
neuroplasticity, 35, 40, 76, 99
nociceptive pain, 21, 41, 127, 129, 152
nociceptor, 24–25, 27, 33
non-modifiable risk factors and chronic pain, 69; age, 70–71; ethnicity and cultural background, 74; for osteoarthritis, 84; gender, 71–72; genetic factors, 72–73; physical and psychological trauma, 75; previous surgery pain, 74; socioeconomic status, 73
Numerical Rating Scale (NRS), 128

occasionalism, 44
osteoporosis, 91–92

Index

pain, 146; acute (see Acute pain); as a learned behaviour, 48; as punishment, 5–6; catastrophizing, 11; chronic (see Chronic pain); clinic, 7–14; congenital insensitivity to, 19; defined, 15–18; during life span, xiii; nerve-related phenomenon, 19; prolong, 42; sensitivity, 72; starting of, 18; transition from acute to chronic, 41
painful diabetic neuropathy (PDN), 82
pathological pain, 20–21
pelvic pain, 85–86
peripheral: neuropathy, 82; sensitization, 32–33, 35, 40
personality assessment: by using projective tests, 136–138; Eysenck Personality Questionnaire-Revised (EPQ-R), 135; Rotter's Locus of Control Scale (LOC), 136
personality disorders, 50
phonophobia, 38
photophobia, 38
physical injury, 42
physical pain, xiii–xiv, 145; causes of, 9; impact of, 13, 56
physiological pain, 18, 20–21, 23; defined, 19; pathway, 24–31
physiotherapists, 3, 13, 62, 109, 126, 140, 160–161, 204

physiotherapy, 7, 30, 156–157, 185, 191–193, 199, 202, 204; sessions, 2–3
post-traumatic stress disorder (PTSD), 49, 75
psychic pain, 31
psychogenic pain, 31, 77
psychological disorders, 22–23, 31, 49, 58, 67, 76
psychological pain, 10, 17, 23; adaptive function of, 19; impact of, 21
psychophysical parallelism, 44
psychosocial assessment of patients, xiv

risk factors: modifiable risk factors (see Modifiable risk factors); non-modifiable (see Non-modifiable risk factors)

Saunders, Dame Cicely, 17
sciatica, 99, 102, 141–142, 154
secondary gains, 48, 54, 115
self-efficacy, 9, 59–61, 104
self-esteem, 60, 75, 86, 112–113, 120, 136
self-management, 148
self-revelation, 202
Selye, Hans, 57
short-lived pain, 95
social interactions and environment role in treatment programme: Dyadic

Adjustment Scale (DAS), 134–135
social pain, 6, 9–10, 17
social therapies for mind treatment: family therapy, 180; (cognitive behavioural transactional process therapy, 182; operant behavioural therapy, 181–182; structural, 181); group therapy, 183–185; marital therapy, 182–183
spiritual pain, 10, 14, 17
stress, 11, 18, 70. See also Chronic pain; daily hassles or chronic, 57; life events, 57; proneness to, 57–58; psychological, 57
stress inoculation therapy (SIT), 173
substance use disorder (SUD), 203
supportive psychotherapeutic methods: control and release of tension, 177; environmental manipulation, 177–178; externalization of interests, 178–180; importance of reassurance, 177; persuasion, 178; ventilation, 176–177

thought-emotion-behaviour combination in chronic pain, 45–48

tolerance to pain, 71–72, 74, 89, 108
total pain, concept of, 9–10, 17
trauma, 21, 59, 70; emotional, 6; extensive, 32; physical, 36, 75; psychological, 36, 75
treatment of chronic pain, pharmacological and interventional methods for, 159; nutrition role in, 162–164; physical activity, 160–161; physical therapy, 160–161; sleep disorders management, 161–162
treatment of mind, therapies for: behaviour (see Behaviour therapies for mind treatment); psychological, 164; social therapies (see Social therapies for mind treatment); supportive psychotherapeutic methods (see Supportive psychotherapeutic methods)

Visual Analogue Scale (VAS), 128
visualization (or imagery), 165–166
Vitamin D deficiency, 92

WHO: health, definition, 189; three-step analgesic ladder, 148–149, 151
Wong-Baker FACES Pain Rating Scale, 128

About the Authors

Dr Vandana V. Prakash is a senior consultant clinical psychologist practising for the past thirty years. She has an MPhil in medical and social psychology from NIMHANS, Bangalore. She has several research papers to her credit and has co-authored chapters on suicidal behaviour in adolescents for various international publications. She has also co-authored *Conquering Pain* (2019). Her next book is about learning disabilities. Dr Prakash is a clinician, researcher, academician and trainer.

Dr Mary Abraham is MD (AIIMS) and DNB anaesthesiology, with thirty-five years of experience in neuroanaesthesiology, pain and palliative care. She is a senior consultant in pain at the Max Multi Speciality Centre, Panchsheel Park, New Delhi. She has several papers to her credit, has contributed chapters in various books and has co-authored *Conquering Pain* (2019). She has organized many conferences and conducted workshops on neuroanaesthesia and pain medicine. She has contributed medical illustrations to various books, including *Managing Chronic Pain*. Dr Abraham is a clinician, researcher and academician.

HarperCollins *Publishers* India

At HarperCollins India, we believe in telling the best stories and finding the widest readership for our books in every format possible. We started publishing in 1992; a great deal has changed since then, but what has remained constant is the passion with which our authors write their books, the love with which readers receive them, and the sheer joy and excitement that we as publishers feel in being a part of the publishing process.

Over the years, we've had the pleasure of publishing some of the finest writing from the subcontinent and around the world, including several award-winning titles and some of the biggest bestsellers in India's publishing history. But nothing has meant more to us than the fact that millions of people have read the books we published, and that somewhere, a book of ours might have made a difference.

As we look to the future, we go back to that one word—a word which has been a driving force for us all these years.

Read.